The Miracle of
GARLIC &
VINEGAR

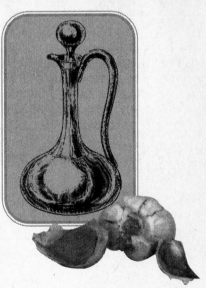

by James Edmond O'Brien

Contents

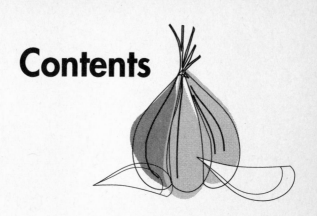

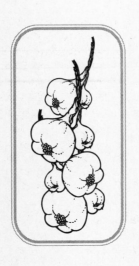

You Are What You Eat

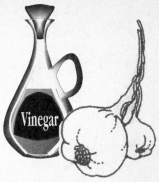

Some foods are more than mere nourishment. They are astonishing healers entwined in history and mystery. Garlic tops that list quite easily. Its folklore dates back thousands of years, and it continues to fascinate us. It's used all over the world in cooking and in natural medicine.

Vinegar, though without the same mystique and written lore, possesses a similarly remarkable range of properties. Other natural wonders like honey, seaweed and a long list of herbs offer extraordinary healing aid as well. They are generally safe and promise a low-cost route to good health.

"When you eat what nature offers, the reward is long life, happiness, health, wealth and prosperity," said Dr. George Blodgett, a physician and nutritionist who lived to the ripe old age of 94, mainly by practicing what he preached.

He recommended these simple rules for good health: Eat a clove of garlic a day, drink two teaspoons of apple cider vinegar in a glass of warm water every morning and evening, and add a teaspoon of honey. If desired, add a drop of lemon juice.

This was his prescription for good health because, he said, his lifelong research demonstrated that these foods supply all of the biochemicals, vitamins and minerals, in the right balance, to sustain life and promote health.

Only in Dr. Blodgett's last years did science begin, grudgingly, to accept that he had been right on target all along.

The Stinking Rose

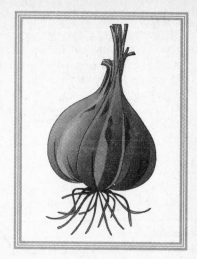

With all of the impressive findings that scientists have made about garlic, it would come as no surprise if we discovered that it truly does repel vampires, just like those Dracula stories report.

Few foods possess as rich a past and as detailed a history. Scientists have already taken garlic seriously enough to study it at some length. And in a remarkable number of instances, they have verified all of the amazing claims handed down through the centuries in folk healers' literature and old wives' tales.

Entire books have been written about this humble-looking bulb by reputable authors. There is even a garlic appreciation society – called, of all things, 'Lovers of the Stinking Rose' – organized to extoll its wonders.

Every year there are festivals held to praise it, where its worshipers swap stories about new uses, favorite recipes and the most effective methods of farming it.

And its success in the marketplace underscores all of this pomp and circumstance. It is the second most popular spice (after pepper) in North America. Think about it... it's in so many of the things we eat – chips, dips, powders, spreads, sauces, flakes, purées and all kinds of concentrates.

And most of all, it tastes so absolutely wonderful. Unfortunately, as with most things worthwhile in life, there's a downside, too. As good as garlic can make foods taste, it can also make us smell very, very bad.

Which brings us to garlic breath. Of course, most of us

could do without that, but the reality is that if everybody in the country ate garlic, none of us would notice it very much. It would be so much a part of all of our lives that it would become, believe it or not, virtually unnoticeable!

That lingering, clinging, all-pervasive odor is created by essential oils in the garlic bulb. These oils enter your bloodstream and circulate for quite a long time – up to several hours.

This is, at one and the same time, the blessing and the curse of garlic, because it is these oils circulating in the bloodstream that makes the garlic work its therapeutic wonders. And while it does that, it produces the characteristic odor. That's because the source of the smell is deep in the bloodstream. Mouthwash, toothbrushing or chewing gum are thus all destined to fail against garlic breath.

You may mask the odor on your breath for a little while – just as long as that minty toothpaste keeps its smell – but that won't outlast the garlic. After that, as you may have discovered through experience, it will come right back, leaking out of the pores of your skin.

Garlic odor on the breath can be controlled by eating fresh parsley. Chewing on a coffee bean or two after consuming the 'stinking rose' also does the trick.

Natural Perfume

Despite its bad breath rap, however, garlic can actually perfume the air. During the process of cooking, the odor of garlic teases the senses with its magical, mouthwatering fragrance. Just walk through any Italian restaurant kitchen and breathe in that garlic aroma that wafts from pots on the stove and casseroles in the oven. It truly is a glorious delight.

All of this tends to overshadow the lighter side of the garlic story. For centuries in Asia and ancient Rome, it has enjoyed a reputation as an aphrodisiac. So far, we have been unable to locate any serious, scientific study that supports that reputation, but it's worth bearing in mind that old wives' tales frequently have more than a grain of truth to them!

Garlic is described in horticultural manuals as a 'culinary herb'. It's a member of the lily

9

family and is very easy to grow at home. The technical Latin name is *allium sativum*, which categorizes garlic as a hardy perennial bulb. It is a first cousin to the family that includes onions, leeks, chives, scallions and shallots. It is grown, harvested and cured. The bulbs form cloves. Naked stalks climb out of the ground, and sometimes, but not always, white flowers form at the tops of these stems. You can harvest it from either the bulb or green shoots – both provide the delicate flavor that you are seeking.

Garlic has been grown for thousands of years all over the world. Horticulturalists say there are dozens, perhaps even hundreds, of different varieties, and there are estimates ranging from a low of 30 to a high of 300 separate strains. Each one offers a unique virtue, but the same flavor and healthful properties are common to all of these strains.

And nothing can quite compare with the wonderful taste of garlic.

Lloyd J. Harris sums it up in his book *The Official Garlic Lover's Handbook*. "The flavor of fresh garlic has not, as yet, been duplicated by any processing techniques that I know of. Because garlic oxidizes so readily when it is cut, commercial products must add other substances such as citric acid and/or oil to preserve them. This alters the wonderfully distinctive flavor of garlic."

Buy It or Grow It

Grocery stores offer a wide variety of very good, whole-clove garlics. Those little cardboard boxes with the clear windows in the center of the carton contain the real thing. When you cook with this, be sure to use all of any single clove you peel and open – it just doesn't keep fresh once it has been exposed to the air.

You can grow it, too. The great medieval king Charlemagne ordered all of his subjects to grow garlic in their gardens, declaring it one of those rare herbs that are "the friend of physicians and the praise of cooks..."

Garlic is remarkably easy for

you to cultivate on your own. If you do decide to go that route, ask the advice of any gardener or nurseryman and follow his instructions faithfully. Remember, though, that the 'fresh' garlic label rarely means that it has just come straight out of the ground. While you can eat freshly pulled garlic, it is actually the drying and curing process that gives it its full and truly distinctive flavor.

Because it's cured, garlic retains its flavor and goodness for many months if you store it properly. The key to a long shelf life is leaving it where air can circulate freely around it. Keep it in a cool and dry place – basements and garages are ideal.

You can braid garlic stems to form bunches that are pleasing to the eye, or you can store them in the types of mesh bags in which you usually find onions, in old nylon stockings or on wire racks.

Other storage methods include dehydrating, puréeing, marinating in vegetable or olive oil and refrigerating. Ironically, of all the storage options, placing whole cloves in the refrigerator is the least effective method of storage. It certainly works, but refrigerators tend to be too damp and cold for long-term preservation. So if you decide to store garlic in those little compartments on the door of the fridge, plan to use it in the very near future.

If you grow garlic at home, dry the bulbs thoroughly for about two weeks in a closet or in the garage or basement. To cure them, trim the roots off, leaving about half an inch of stem. Then braid or tie the bulbs together in bunches and hang them from rafters or herb-drying stands for two weeks to a month.

After that, they're ready to eat. If you have more than you can conveniently consume in short order, store as described above.

They Know Their Garlic

Gilroy, CA, bills itself as the 'Garlic Capital of the World'. It boasts a $54 million-a-year garlic industry in a town with a population of only 27,400.

Humorist Will Rogers described Gilroy as, "the only town in America where you can marinate a steak by hanging it on the clothesline," in reference to the pungent odor that pervades the city.

Ninety percent of the garlic

consumed in the 50 states is shipped through Gilroy for processing and packaging, much of it grown within a radius of 90 miles of the town.

The good folks in Gilroy have written a book called *The Complete Garlic Lovers' Cookbook*. It includes recipes and pointers such as those below on how to spot, treat and eat garlic.

Garlic in the Kitchen

Knowing the correct **technique for peeling garlic will save you time and energy: If you only want to use a few cloves, press them between the thumb and forefinger to loosen the skin first, then place on a cutting board and press down on them with the flat side of a heavy kitchen knife.**

For larger quantities, drop cloves into boiling water for a minute and drain, after which they'll peel easily. Five seconds in a microwave oven achieves the same effect.

Please note, peeling is not always mandatory. You can try cooking unpeeled cloves in a hot pan; this will protect the garlic meat from burning, and the skin will slip off when the garlic is soft.

And if you're going to cook the garlic in a soup or stew, why bother going to the trouble of peeling? The flavor will reach the dish, and you can throw out the garlic later. There are techniques for containing the fragrance left on your hands after peeling and chopping garlic, as well. For one thing, wear rubber gloves while you're working. You could also rub your fingers with salt and lemon juice afterward, then rinse with cold water.

The Gilroy garlic experts say the best solution they have found is to clasp your fingers around the bowl of a stainless steel teaspoon under running water for a few moments. A chemical reaction takes place that does, indeed, eliminate the odor from your fingers.

To purée garlic, peel and run through a blender or food processor. Put the purée in a jar and add a teaspoon of lemon juice or some olive oil for each ½ pint of purée. Refrigerate for at least a day.

If you want to dehydrate it, slice the cloves into ⅛-inch slices and lay them out on a cheesecloth to dry in the sun. You can also use a gas oven. Leave them until they turn into little chips that snap. Then you can store them inside a tightly sealed jar in a cool cupboard for years. Do not refrigerate. Use them in soups, salads and sauces.

Marinating garlic is a snap. Slice and place in a jar of extra virgin olive oil in the refrigerator. You may add herbs if you wish. It is important to use extra virgin grade olive oil because lesser grades will congeal under refrigeration.

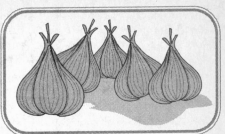

Garlic in History

Garlic is mentioned in the earliest recorded texts and played an important role in the cultures of the great nations of antiquity that flourished around the Mediterranean, such as Mesopotamia, Sumeria, Assyria, Egypt and Persia, as well as India and China.

In fact, researchers have found references to garlic in Chinese texts dating back as far as 2,000 years before Christ. That means civilization has been familiar with garlic and its uses as a foodstuff and healing agent for at least 4,000 years.

Interestingly, the ancient Chinese thought garlic was especially good for purifying water and preventing food poisoning from improperly prepared meat and fish. That usage is confirmed by modern scientific findings, which have shown that the germ-killing properties in garlic can preserve meat, keeping it fresh and edible two to four times longer than meat not treated with garlic.

Yale University scholars have recently unearthed Babylonian tablets from the year 1700 B.C. – almost 4,000 years ago – listing recipes that strongly feature garlic and onions. And archaeologists have found illustrations of a garlic clove in the tomb of the pharaoh Tutankhamen.

Many historians suspect that garlic first took root, so to speak, some place in Asia – maybe Siberia – and was brought through Asia Minor to the Fertile Crescent, the Red Sea and the regions surrounding the fertile delta of the river

Nile. From there it was probably spread to Europe by seagoing traders, and the rest, as they say, is history.

According to the Talmud, the authority on Jewish law and tradition, the eating of garlic satisfied hunger, kept the body warm, brightened the complexion, killed parasites in the body, removed jealousy and promoted love. Interestingly, the Talmud recommends garlic as an aphrodisiac and suggests eating it on Friday – the night traditionally set aside for marital lovemaking, according to writer Alexandra Hicks.

In ancient Greece, Hippocrates, the father of modern medicine, used garlic for treating infections, wounds and intestinal disorders – not to mention a reportedly mean lamb stew and an outstanding vegetable soup. Roman legionnaires attributed their strength, courage and stamina to garlic and took it with them as they conquered the world – thus spreading its use and cultivation everywhere they went.

Since then, garlic has enjoyed a huge importance in the cooking and cultures of Mediterranean countries such as Italy, Spain and Turkey, and on the North African coast, Morocco and Tunisia.

Curiously enough, in England and eventually in America, there was quite a bit of resistance to garlic, but the bulb has finally made it big. Look at the numbers: More than 200 million pounds of garlic are grown commercially in this country every year.

Demons and Demigods

It may strike you as somewhat strange, but there is even evidence that garlic has been given a demi-god status and worshiped – as well as being denounced as a demon – during various periods in history. I am not suggesting for a moment that we take our enthusiasm for garlic to that kind of length, but it does emphasize the intense effect garlic can have on people's hearts and minds, as well as their palates!

Let's take a closer look at the myths or superstitions, if you will, because a startling amount of these are being confirmed scientifically today.

The world still marvels at the pyramids at Giza, built by the ancient Egyptians as a stunning testament to their ingenuity and monument to their kings. Inscriptions inside these structures in the Valley of the Kings indicate that the workers who built them subsisted largely on onions, garlic and radishes, and that to them they were more than mere foodstuffs.

The Egyptians credited these foods, especially garlic, with magical and medicinal powers responsible for the physical stamina and spiritual integrity necessary for the workers to complete their backbreaking tasks. And apparently the workers subscribed to the same theory, because when the supplies of garlic ran out, they went on strike – something virtually unheard of in that day and age.

An Egyptian holy book, the *Codex Ebers*, was discovered in 1878 by the distinguished German archaeologist George Ebers. It dates from about 1550 B.C. and lists more than 800 therapeutic formulas in use at the time. Twenty-two of them were based on garlic and these were said to heal headaches, heart problems, body weakness, human bites, intestinal parasites, throat tumors and any problems relating to childbirth and the menstrual cycle.

The Bible tells how the Hebrews considered garlic to be a magic talisman against evil spirits, protecting people from the diseases brought on by angry demons.

In ancient Palestine, garlic was believed to promote fertility in women having difficulty conceiving children. It was also firmly recommended as protection against the 'evil eye' – just as, many centuries later, it was reported to protect against vampires and werewolves.

The prophet of Islam, Mohammed, recommended garlic as an antidote to the stings and bites of poisonous insects, snakes and other animals. The ancient Greeks, on the other hand, used garlic talismans to guard against the mischief of the beautiful Nereids, malicious, half-divine, half-human

15

nymphs who tried to lead wives and mothers-to-be astray.

Throughout the civilizations of ancient Rome, early India and China, garlic was considered potent medicine, as it was throughout medieval Europe.

And on into modern times, garlic has maintained its place as a favorite food and valued medicine. This is particularly so in the south of France (in a region called Provence, where the ancient city of Avignon is located), in Italy and in Spain.

The strangest belief about garlic originated in Eastern Europe, where people used it to repel vampires. We may chuckle at the notion now, but it wasn't all that long ago that they lived in mortal fear that their lifeblood would be sucked from them as they slept.

They hung garlands of garlic around their necks and in bunches in the doorways and windows of their homes to keep them safe from vampires.

They also believed that once they caught a vampire and killed it, garlic could help keep it dead – hence the literary tradition, carried on in countless Hollywood horror flicks, of stuffing garlic in a vampire's mouth and filling its coffin with whole cloves before burial. This,

of course, presupposes catching the vampire and killing it, either with a silver bullet or burying a stake in its heart.

The Americas

Native Americans used garlic as a charm to rid young maidens of unwanted suitors. South American revolutionary San Martin, who led the fight for independence of Argentina, Chile and Peru in the 19th century, had his men, horses and mules sniff and chew garlic to combat altitude sickness as they crossed the towering Andes mountain range.

In Cuba, 13 cloves of garlic at the end of a string worn around the neck for a period of 13 days, no more, no less, was regarded as a surefire way to keep jaundice away. For best results, arise in the middle of the night of the 13th day, said the tradition, go to the intersection of two streets, take off the garlic necklace, fling it behind you and run home without looking back. If you were to look over your shoulder, a bogeyman would hunt you down.

Lloyd J. Harris, author of *The Book of Garlic*, says the

history of garlic makes one point abundantly clear: "...that garlic has always been a 'people's' food and remedy (magical and medical); and where the people loved it most, the upper classes (priests, kings, aristocrats and politicians) created taboos against it. The people worshiped it anyway."

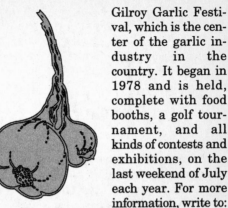

Modern America and high technology are helping overcome this snooty view of garlic. The reason for that may be simple. As we'll see, it is found in present-day medical literature.

Garlic Festivals

For thousands of years, the people of the world have celebrated garlic with feasting, festivals and celebration. Now we do it all over America as well, although without question, California is the garlic-festival capital.

There is, of course, the granddaddy of them all, the Gilroy Garlic Festival, which is the center of the garlic industry in the country. It began in 1978 and is held, complete with food booths, a golf tournament, and all kinds of contests and exhibitions, on the last weekend of July each year. For more information, write to: Gilroy Garlic Festival, P.O. Box 2311, Gilroy, CA 95020.

Smaller festivals throughout the country are held in Berkeley, CA (at a restaurant called Chez Panisse); Nahcotta, WA (at the Ark restaurant); Camp Verde, AZ, and Denver, CO. Contact the chamber of commerce in each city for details. International events take place in Takko Machi, Japan; Poilene and Arleux, France; Sudbury, Ont., Canada; and Motecelli, Italy, as well as in Czechoslovakia, Germany, and the Isle of Wight.

The Fitchburg Garlic Festival is held at an Italian church, Madonna of the Holy Rosary, in Fitchburg, MA, every June. For information, write to Rev. Pat Biscardi at the church.

The Great Healer

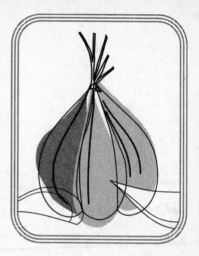

Here's where we go beyond mere character and ancestry to delve into the reasons why we truly can apply the term 'wonder food' to garlic.

Healing power, medicinal value, a cure for what ails you, call it what you want, garlic is the real thing.

"Thousands of years of folklore couldn't all be wrong, and laboratory analysis has proven that it is true," says Dr. Victor Gurewich, director of the Tufts University Vascular Laboratory at St. Elizabeth's Hospital in Boston. He and his colleagues conducted extensive tests on garlic and onions that showed their amazing ability to lower total cholesterol and protect against heart attacks and hardening of the arteries.

Scientific understanding of the natural gift of garlic has come a long way in less than a century. Around the year 1900, garlic ointments, com-

presses and compounds were the common treatment of choice. Military surgeons in World War I, who did not have modern antibiotics available to them, used it to cleanse wounds, combat infections and prevent and treat gangrene. It worked so well that British surgeons still relied on it extensively during World War II, even though antibiotics were available by then.

Even today in the former Soviet Union, garlic is still used to kill bacteria and fight infections. Some tests even show it is more effective than antibiotics for specific types of bacterial infection termed 'gram negative'. Throughout Europe this has earned garlic the nick-

18

name 'Russian penicillin'.

Since the 1940s, scientific investigation has proven garlic possesses a stunning array of medicinal properties. Investigators say that it:

- **Acts as an antiseptic**
- **Fights infection**
- **Contains chemicals that prevent cancer**
- **Thins the blood, reducing clotting in high-risk heart patients**
- **Lowers blood pressure**
- **Reduces cholesterol**
- **Controls triglycerides**
- **Stimulates the immune system**
- **Prevents and relieves chronic bronchitis**
- **Acts as a decongestant and expectorant**

Heart Disease

The National Library of Medicine, in Bethesda, MD, contains more than 125 scientific papers written about the medicinal value of garlic since 1983 alone.

Garlic has an amazingly high sulfur content, and it is this, experts say, that makes all the difference.

In most cases, they say you need merely eat a clove or two a day, cut up in salads and soups, to enjoy its healing properties.

Let's examine some of these findings in greater detail.

Heart disease is the leading killer of Americans, accounting for nearly one in two deaths in this country every year. Studies show garlic can reduce those numbers and protect you and your family.

Garlic prevents heart attacks and strokes by controlling the key variables of high cholesterol, high triglycerides, high blood pressure and atherosclerosis – the deadly process of plaque formation and fat deposits inside the arteries. These factors create blockages in the circulatory system that ultimately can choke blood flow to the heart muscle or brain.

The simplest explanation for this is that garlic thins the blood. Dr. George Blodgett spent six years doing laboratory research back in the 1920s and saw microscopic evidence of garlic's workings. "It dissolves fat particles and out-of-place blood clots and keeps them in suspension until they can be eliminated through the bowel – as long as it's circulating and your body's excreting it, it can't hurt you. The stuff works, and it beats me why we insist on fancier, more expensive prescription medicines when nature already provides what we need."

Dr. Blodgett used garlic as a heart medication during his nearly 70-year practice, because it worked. That's all he cared about. "What else do you need to know?" he said.

An esteemed German physician, Dr. Hans Reuter, of Cologne, Germany, reported clinical studies in the mid-to-late 1970s proving the effectiveness of garlic against heart disease on three fronts: controlling cholesterol, blood pres-

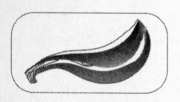

sure and fatty deposits in the arteries. He recommended just one to three cloves daily. Simply add it to soup or salad.

But modern medicine works in mysterious ways, and for reasons not readily apparent, it is highly resistant to change. Conservatism and caution seems built into the profession.

With rare exception, physicians have been highly skeptical of Dr. Reuter's findings, despite his high standing in the academic community.

Lowering Cholesterol

Investigators in India, Bulgaria, Libya and Japan have produced some powerful scientific evidence supporting garlic's role in warding off heart disease. American scientists, I'm sorry to admit, tend to be insular, to say the least – some critics might say self-centered and egotistical – and look down their noses at any work carried out by their non-American colleagues.

They also discount what they call 'anecdotal reports' or empirical evidence – such as the decades of case histories that Dr. Blodgett could produce. Unless the evidence comes from what are called controlled scientific trials, they insist such reports simply don't count.

Happily, a few suspected that where there was smoke there might well be fire.

One of them was Dr. David Kritchevsky, now associate

director of the Wistar Institute in Philadelphia.

"I was doing postdoctoral work in Switzerland," he says, "when I discovered that my landlady – a 66-year-old woman who looked 44 and acted 22 – attributed her good health to the fact that she ate a clove of garlic chopped up in her salad every single night."

He was inclined, at first, to dismiss her report as superstitious nonsense, but he discovered that other Europeans offered similar witness. That prompted him to begin a serious investigation into garlic's possible impact on heart disease.

The Evidence

All Kritchevsky's experiments demonstrated that rabbits fed a diet that included garlic oil had 10 percent lower blood cholesterol levels and between 15 and 45 percent less fat in their arteries than rabbits that did not consume the garlic oil. Subsequent studies confirmed that the effect held true in rats, as well.

Armed with this evidence, Kritchevsky then reviewed scientific literature from around the world and concluded that garlic does exactly what his landlady claimed. But he still had reservations. "The trouble is, the dosage required for humans seems pretty high," he says.

Other studies have laid his fears to rest.

The prestigious British medical journal *The Lancet* published a study by two Indian cardiologists that showed that raw garlic will, indeed, protect you from heart disease.

You don't have to change anything else in your diet, mind you; all you have to do is add garlic. Of course, the greater care you take to observe a low-fat, high-fiber diet, the better off you will be. But Drs. Bordia and Bansal of the Department of Medicine at R.N.T. Medical College in Udaipur, India, found that garlic controls cholesterol so effectively that it even overcomes the cardiotoxic effects of butter fat.

In their controlled experiments they gave their subjects a meal that included a ¼-pound serving of butter. Just as they expected, blood cholesterol levels soared. They repeated the experiment, but this time they added 50 grams of raw garlic to the butter (equal to about two cloves). The results were truly astonishing. The garlic lowered blood cholesterol by more than 25 percent from the pre-meal fasting level.

Blood Clots

Even after consuming that very large, highly imprudent, amount of butter, the addition of garlic had left these patients better off than before they had eaten. The garlic also counteracted a tendency for blood to clot in unwanted ways after a high-fat meal.

The authors wrote, "It is obvious that garlic has a very significant protective action against *hyperlipidemia* (high cholesterol) and blood coagulation changes, which are normal after fat ingestion." And all this without the high cost and risk of the prescription drugs that are so frequently used to lower cholesterol.

The report went on to explain that garlic carried few of these risks and was perfectly safe to use on a long-term basis. It would be particularly helpful, it said, in preventing symptoms of *alimentary* hyperlipidemia (the tendency to turn digested food into cholesterol) in people at risk of developing arteriosclerosis. This high-risk group includes those who have diabetes, high blood pressure or a family history of stroke and heart disease. And that means, all told, about 170 million Americans.

Studies published in the *American Journal of Clinical Nutrition* verify these findings.

Other human tests showed that about ⅙ of a cup of fresh garlic juice every day drastically reduced blood cholesterol, from an average reading of 305 to 218, in just two months.

Still other studies showed garlic has an amazing ability to discriminate between 'good' HDL and 'bad' LDL cholesterol. LDL increases heart disease risk by promoting fat deposits inside the arteries; they are, figuratively, dump trucks in your blood that drop loads of fat along the inside walls of your arteries. HDL is just the opposite and protects you; it is, figuratively, an earth mover, scooping loads of fat from inside your arteries and hauling it away to the liver and bowel, where it can be eliminated.

"We found that garlic or onions in amounts that you'd consider normal to eat, raised the level of HDL cholesterol just as effectively as daily, vigorous exercise," says Dr. Gurewich.

Dr. Myung Chi of Lincoln University in Missouri has confirmed this effect of garlic in his own experiments and believes it may also prove effective in relieving high blood pressure.

And that's not all. The Japanese, who seem to come up with something clever every day, apparently approach the field of garlic no differently than they do the world of automobiles or electronics. They have developed a garlic extract concentrate that eliminates that bothersome odor while retaining all of its wonderfully beneficial properties. They call it *kyolic*. And it works.

In 1987, Dr. Benjamin Lau at Loma Linda University in California used kyolic in a heart disease experiment with dramatic effects. They found that a gram of kyolic (the equivalent of about nine cloves of garlic) lowered total cholesterol about 10 percent on average, but as much as 50 percent in some individuals, and it lowered LDL cholesterol levels in 70 percent of the volunteers in the study.

What's more, garlic actually dissolves life-threatening blood clots. Dr. Martyn Bailey of Georgetown University in Washington, D.C., has produced laboratory evidence that a chemical in garlic called *adenosine* blocks the production of a blood compound named *fibronolytic*, which makes blood sticky and causes clotting.

To put it another way, this means that garlic thins the blood. And adenosine isn't the only weapon in garlic's arsenal, says chemistry professor Dr. Eric Block of the Albany Medical College. By teaming adenosine with a chemical Dr. Block discovered called *ajoene* (which is what you'd call a medical marvel, because it also has antibiotic properties and promotes wound healing), garlic can give untimely blood clots a knockout punch.

Block says quite bluntly that "as an *antithrombotic* agent (clot buster), ajoene is at least as potent as aspirin." And aspirin has been recognized as one of the most effective anticoagulants, or blood thinners, going. Block's animal experiments show that a single dose of ajoene will shut down platelet aggregation (unwanted clotting) by 100 percent and keep it that way for 24 hours.

All of these researchers stress firmly that garlic has ab-

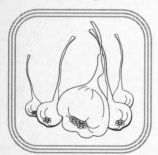

solutely no side effects of any kind. The only risk you can possibly run as a confirmed consumer of garlic is that of offending your friends. And kyolic can eliminate that hazard if it concerns you.

But that's just the tip of the iceberg when it comes to the healing powers of garlic.

Infection Fighter

Garlic kills germs. In 1944, chemist Chester Cavallito identified the smelly compound in garlic, called *allicin*, and demonstrated that it was a highly effective antibiotic. Other tests have confirmed that garlic is an even more powerful germ-killer than either penicillin or tetracycline.

The list of microbes that garlic can slay includes botulism, tuberculosis, diarrhea, staph, dysentery, pneumonia, sepsis and typhoid. Reports list 72 separate bugs garlic can bump off; bacteria, yeast, fungus (tuberculosis is the best-known fungal infection); parasites and protozoa all yield to garlic.

Cooking neutralizes allicin, so you need raw garlic for its antibiotic properties. Many doctors will tell you that a compress of mashed garlic can keep cuts and wounds clean and free of infection.

There are some reports that applying garlic directly to skin cancers makes the tumor disappear within weeks.

The most significant recent discovery is that garlic

also kills viruses. This has potentially enormous significance.

It means that the next time you feel a cold or flu coming on, add a few cloves of raw garlic to your chicken soup and you'll not only feel better for a while, you'll beat the illness outright.

"If you do it early enough, you may not even get sick," says Dr. James North, chief of microbiology at Brigham Young University in Provo, UT.

Virus Killer

North conducted experiments showing garlic as a potent virus killer, and the implications of his findings are stunning. Not only do common ailments such as the cold come within garlic's medicinal reach, but more serious diseases such as herpes and polio do, too.

His data shows garlic extract kills with near 100 percent effectiveness:

- **Human rhinovirus, which causes colds**
- **Parainfluenza 3, a common flu and respiratory virus**

- **Herpes simplex 1, which causes fever blisters**
- **Herpes simplex 2, responsible for genital herpes**

In addition, garlic has killed the polio virus with 90 percent effectiveness and proven capable of tackling the deadly HIV or AIDS virus. Once scientists identify the active virus-killing chemical in garlic, they may be able to make a concentrated pill for treating these very serious ailments.

Nobody is saying garlic cures cancer. The reason I'm stating that is because the American Cancer Society hunts down people who use the word cure in connection with cancer as if they were witches. Having said that, let's take a look at the evidence that garlic's astonishing healing touch extends even to the 'Big C'.

Back in 1952, Russian scientists used garlic extracts against human tumors. Colon cancer – one of the most common forms of the disease – may be particularly susceptible to garlic.

Dr. Michael Wargovich of the University of Texas, Anderson Hospital and Tumor Institute, has found that mice treated with a chemical in garlic are 75 percent less likely

25

to develop malignancies in the large bowel. The National Cancer Institute is taking these findings seriously enough to investigate the matter further and currently places garlic high on its list of 'chemopreventives', which are substances that block carcinogens.

Bladder cancer may not stand a chance against it, either. Animal experiments by Dr. Lau demonstrated that garlic extract (kyolic) inhibited this deadly malignancy.

Chinese researchers, together with scientists at Cornell University and the National Cancer Institute, say garlic, as well as onions and scallions, can dramatically cut your risk of stomach cancer. The more you eat, the lower your risk, and depending on how much you are prepared to eat, you can almost triple your protection.

Diabetes

The U.S. Department of Agriculture's Human Nutrition Center in Beltsville, MD, has demonstrated that the herb can reduce not only levels of blood fat, but blood sugar, too, at the same time increasing the level of insulin in the blood. That spells one thing: better diabetes control.

Dr. Tarig Abdullah of the Akbar Clinic and Research Institute in Panama City, FL, has produced dramatic evidence that glorious garlic revs up the body's natural immune system.

He and nine other volunteers ate either raw garlic or kyolic extract. He then drew the volunteers' blood and the blood of a control group made up of people who had not eaten any garlic. The next step was to extract key immune system components such as white blood cells and killer cells (a type of white blood cell that attacks and kills invaders). They were mixed in a lab dish with cancer cells. The result was astonishing – killer cells from the garlic eaters destroyed from 140 percent to 160 percent more cancer cells than did blood from the non-garlic eaters.

Abdullah ate large amounts of garlic himself, as many as 10 to 15 cloves a day, but is convinced you can obtain a protective effect from smaller doses. He also believes his finding may be of extreme importance to AIDS treatment. He also reports that he has not had a cold since he started eating a couple of garlic cloves a day back in 1973.

Better Living, Naturally

The chemical breakdown of garlic provides some real insight into its many medicinal talents. It is a mineral- and vitamin-rich food, but it is the especially high concentration of sulfur compounds (*allyl sulphides*) that truly set it apart.

According to analysis by the U.S. Department of Agriculture, a single clove of garlic contains:

- 7 calories
- .31 gm protein
- .01 gm fat
- 1.5 gm carbohydrate
- 1.4 mg calcium
- 10 mg phosphorus
- .07 mg iron
- .9 mg sodium
- 26 mg potassium
- .01 mg B1
- .004 mg B2
- .02 mg niacin
- .75 mg vitamin C

Alliin, allinase and *allicin* by name are the big three for you to particularly remember. These are sulphur compounds. They have drawn the attention of serious scientists since the illustrious Louis Pasteur pointed to the antiseptic properties of garlic in 1858.

In the 1940s, Dr. Arthur Stoll, a Nobel Prize-winning scientist, discovered alliin, which he showed to be the 'parent' compound of the germ-fighting process. It must be broken down before garlic gives off its odor and before its antibiotic properties are released. The enzyme allinase, also present in garlic, starts the reaction. All it takes is cutting or crushing the garlic clove and the two combine to produce allicin. For science buffs, the technical name is *allylthiosulphinic acid diallyl disulphide*. This breaks down diallyl disulphide (the stinky stuff) and allythiosulphinate, the medicinal essence.

Even though standard antibiotics are a bit stronger than what garlic provides, U.S. researchers have noted that garlic is more effective against certain germs called gram negative organisms than conventional medications.

Garlic is also loaded with selenium, an important trace element, and Dr. Gerhard Schrauzer of the University of California at San Diego says it offers protection against cancer and atherosclerosis and normalizes blood pressure. It is also an antioxidant, a chemical that neutralizes harsh compounds called free radicals, which accelerate the aging process, so this may account for the antiaging power of garlic.

Germanium is a relatively recent discovery – like selenium, it is also a trace element – and it is thought to offer significant health benefits, because it stimulates oxygen circulation throughout the human body. Garlic contains this trace element, too.

There's even more evidence of garlic's entry into modern medicine and nutrition. Dr. William Castelli, director of the world famous Framingham Study on cholesterol and heart disease, includes garlic on his list of foods that contribute to the prevention of heart disease.

Sometimes it seems as though almost every day there is a new study on garlic mentioned in the media.

"I've given up trying to keep up with it all," writes Lloyd J. Harris in *The Official Garlic Lover's Handbook*. What's encouraging for those who believe in garlic's healing benefits, he says, is that more and more of the studies mentioned in the press are by Americans.

And there is a legion of everyday complaints for which garlic can also provide a cure. For pain, it can be taken mashed, as a tincture, or as an oil, on wounds, abscesses or on stubborn skin infections, although it is strong, so those with sensitive skin should be careful. It can cause blistering.

Also effective is a garlic and water enema, known to promote a speedy recovery from amoebic dysentery. This is used widely in Mexico and in the countries of Central America.

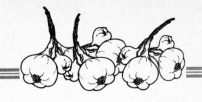

Asthma Fighter

In her book *Herbal Medicine*, Dr. Dian Dincin Buchman, a prominent natural medicine authority, recommends a garlic syrup for asthma that has been in her family for years.

The dosage is 1 tsp with or without water every 15 minutes until the spasm is controlled. Afterward, give the patient 1 tsp every two to three hours for the rest of the day.

Here's the recipe:

Take ½ pound peeled garlic buds, add equal amounts vinegar and distilled water to cover the buds; ½ pint glycerine and 1½ pounds of honey.

Put peeled garlic, vinegar and water in a wide-mouthed jar, close tightly and shake well. Let it stand in a cool place for four or five days, shaking twice daily. Add the glycerine, shake the jar and let stand one more day. Strain and blend in the honey.

Store in a cool place.

'Green' Garlic

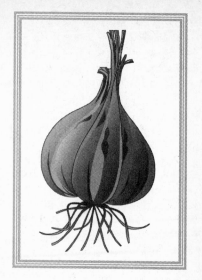

When we speak of the word 'green' in reference to garlic, we're not talking about the color of the bulb – although it can be green – but rather its environmental friendliness. Garlic is a great natural insecticide, capable of ridding houses, gardens, lawns, farms, pets and trees of pests without the harshness and toxicity of chemicals.

The issue of 'green consumerism', using products that don't harm the environment, is shaping into one of the most pressing concerns of the 1990s. Our reliance on plastics and other throwaway materials, the endless stockpiling of refuse and waste materials, and the use of chemicals for everything from washing floors to fueling rockets, is quite literally endangering the existence of our planet.

Huge forests in Europe and North America are withering, lakes are dying and weather patterns are changing – mostly as a result of pollution.

We can wage war for the earth's survival in tiny ways in our own homes and daily lives with the products we buy, with the packaging we insist on, and with the compounds we choose for what seem to be the most simple of tasks.

Take insect repellents, for example. There is no question that those products we use around our homes contribute to pollution. The U.S. and other nations have phased out DDT because of the health horrors it can cause. But instead of seeking natural alternatives, the pros have gone out in search of 'safe' chemicals. The new pesticides are organophosphorous compounds and the *Journal of the American*

Medical Association has stated that while they don't stay in the environment – or the human body – as long as DDT, they're more poisonous.

In its small way, garlic can help you avoid exposure to these horrid compounds. While no one claims that it can solve the pollution crisis, every little bit helps. Garlic, quite simply, kills bugs. Mosquitoes, including those carrying yellow fever and encephalitis, drop dead in its presence. Along

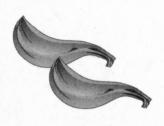

the way, it doesn't hurt people, the soil, the water or the air.

David Greenstock, vice-chairman of The Henry Doubleday Research Association in England, has produced a garlic emulsion that kills malarial mosquitoes that have developed an immunity to DDT. Here are some 'kill' figures to show how garlic solvents work against other pests:

- 87 percent of fire-worm infestation
- 83 percent of cockchafer larvae
- 91 percent of mole crickets
- 82 percent of grey field slugs
- 95 percent of onion fly larvae
- 98 percent of cabbage white caterpillars

Natural Crop Protection

A laboratory experiment produced some especially admirable results against the pea weevil, killing 87 percent of them, Lloyd J. Harris reports in *The Book of Garlic*. This is an insect related to the boll weevil, known to decimate cotton crops, and which many American growers claim requires DDT.

Greenstock has clearly demonstrated that while garlic 'kills bugs dead', it is completely safe and harmless to livestock, wildlife and birds. If anything, veterinarians believe garlic improves the health of animals. (To find out how garlic can help your pets, turn to Garlic, Vinegar & Your Pets, Pg. 81.)

For these reasons, it is standard practice for organic gardeners today to border their plantings with rows of garlic and spray their crops with a garlic solution.

The same should go for you at home: If you are growing just a few herbs or tomatoes, or are raising a more extensive vegetable garden or an orchard of fruit trees, plant some garlic in among your crops, horticulturalists recommend. It will repel the pests and leave you with something else tasty to eat at the end of the growing season – not a heightened risk of cancer some time in the future, which is a real threat from some chemical sprays.

The way it works is simple: The same mechanisms in garlic that kill germs in people also seem to hit insects hard and keep them away from plants. Some researchers say garlic can inhibit protein synthesis in larvae, killing them. Others say it interferes with their breathing process.

Here is David Greenstock's formula for a safe bug spray, as reported by Lloyd J. Harris, publisher of Aris Books:

"Take 3 oz of chopped garlic and let soak in 2 tsp (50 cc) of mineral oil for 24 hours. Then slowly add a pint of water in which ¼ oz of oil-based soap (Palmolive) has been dissolved, and stir well. Strain liquid through fine gauze and store in china or glass container to prevent a reaction with metals. Use it in a dilution of one part solution to 20 parts of water to begin with, then one to 100 thereafter. Apply to plants as spray.

"This is a simple preparation, effective and nontoxic. My wife and I have used it, and we saved a maple sapling from certain death by caterpillar and aphid infestation."

Common Varieties of Garlic

Chilean, while obviously grown in South America, is also found in Japan, Formosa, India and Spain. The bulbs are white and flat and resemble a tangerine in shape and clove arrangement. The color of the cloves is dark pink to wine.

Chileno garlic is a variation on Creole with larger cloves.

Creole is common in Mexico and South America. The plant resembles the late garlic, except it is taller and lighter in color. The skin covering the cloves is dark pink.

Early garlic has broader leaves than the late type and they're light to pale green in color. This strain often displays purplish veins in the skin.

Egyptian is tall and fast growing. It produces large, white bulbs that contain a lot of small cloves in white sheaths.

Elephant garlic is an extremely mild form of garlic that has begun to find its way onto many supermarket shelves. The bulb is approximately the size of a tennis ball.

Italian is grown in Louisiana and in other subtropical parts of the country. Its pink or purplish cloves are stronger in flavor and smaller than the Creole, which is also grown in Louisiana.

The garlic bulbs of this strain are not unlike the artichoke in appearance. The cloves, which are arranged just like artichoke leaves, have thin-layered skins that come off easily. Its leaves are lighter green than those of the Creole.

Continued on Pg. 34

Late garlic has a reputation for keeping a long time. The narrow, upright, dark green leaves and the white sheath surrounding the clove distinguish late garlic from other varieties. The clove ranges in color from light pink to deep red.

Rocambole. Sometimes called 'serpent garlic' because of the coiled shape of its looping green stems, the bulbs are smaller in size than those of plain garlic, although they are equally as pungent. The baby bulbs that form after the flowers fade can be eaten fresh or pickled.

Silverskin is the name given to many garlic strains which have that familiar white outer covering. This is the basic white garlic that many nurseries offer to the would-be gardener/cultivator. It grows well all across the U.S.

Spanish Rojo (Red). This powerfully flavored variety originated in Spain, hence the name. It is very tolerant to drought.

The Gilroy experts suggest starting with the amounts below, which they admit are on the low side. As your tastes change, you may wish to add more:

For meats: Use ⅛ to ¼ tsp of garlic powder or 1½ to 2 tsp of garlic salt or two to three cloves of fresh garlic for every two pounds of meat.

Sauces: Use ⅛ to ¼ tsp of garlic powder or two cloves of fresh garlic for three cups of sauce.

Soups: Add ⅛ tsp of garlic powder or two cloves of fresh garlic.

Pickled foods: Add ⅛ to ¼ tsp of dehydrated, chopped or minced garlic, or two to three cloves fresh.

Relishes: Add ⅛ tsp dehydrated minced garlic or two cloves fresh to two pints of chutney or relish.

Vinegar Power Is Mineral Power

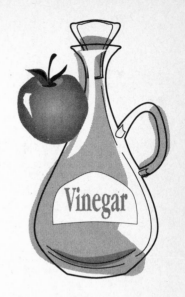

It's an odd coincidence that another common food item – vinegar – with a reputation for smelling odd, could also be so good for you.

For optimum good health and longevity, the experts recommend a glass of water with two teaspoonfuls of apple cider vinegar mixed in, at least twice a day. And they suggest that it's much better to drink the potion once before every meal, every morning on awakening and before going to sleep at night. That's because there are 22 minerals essential for human health, and apple cider vinegar contains 19 of these minerals in exactly the right amounts.

The main benefits from this inexpensive health tonic (which costs less than a penny a day) is a strong and regular heartbeat, a cast-iron digestive tract that nothing can disturb, a pair of kidneys that will never quit, and "freedom from all this allergy business," according to one doctor.

Shortly before his death, my friend Dr. Blodgett gave me a copy of his treasured book, *Folk Medicine, A Vermont Doctor's Guide to Good Health*, by D.C. Jarvis, MD.

Dr. Jarvis was a dyed-in-the-wool physician, ophthalmologist and otolaryngologist, as well as an enthusiast of the ways of folk medicine as they developed in the harsh and hauntingly beautiful climes of his native Vermont. In his own practice, he employed the methods that struck him as most sensible; those that worked stayed in his bag of tricks and those that were not effective, he discarded. Wise Dr. Jarvis was completely convinced that apple cider vinegar could make any living thing healthier. For everyone who sought a more enjoyable, lengthier life, he said, it was an absolute must.

And it all boiled down to one very simple word...

Potassium

That's because folk medicine practitioners, like Jarvis, believe that potassium is the most important of all of the minerals that are necessary for good health. "It is so essential to the life of every living thing that without it there would be no life," Jarvis wrote.

In the last five to 10 years, orthodox medical researchers all over the world have proven the importance of potassium in a number of ways, thus endorsing the findings of the country doctor from New England. Dr. Louis Tobian of the University of Minnesota School of Medicine in Minneapolis, conducted a number of important experiments, which clearly demonstrated that a proper potassium intake can dramatically reduce the symptoms in patients suffering from heartbeat irregularities by well in excess of 50 percent. It will also ensure that every single chemical reaction in the body works at its best. Other studies conducted in a number of centers have shown that nerve and muscle functions throughout the entire human body can suffer severely when the sodium-potassium balance is off.

One fundamental fact all doctors know today is that potassium counteracts the damaging effects of sodium and prevents high blood pressure. It stops unwanted fluid retention and regulates the body's water balance. It normalizes the heart rhythm and works in cells to keep sodium in check.

Dr. Tobian recommends eating a banana and a potato or grapefruit every day to make sure that you get all the potassium your body needs. They are very low in fat and high in fiber. What's more, they have so few calories that they can be eaten without worrying about weight gain.

To get all of the potassium that your body should ideally

have every day, you cannot find a better source than vinegar, writes Jarvis – and apple cider vinegar is the best kind.

Dr. Blodgett believed there is something that occurs in the vinegar that makes the potassium more effective than if it comes from any other source. There are two reasons for that. First, other minerals in the vinegar activate and 'potentiate' the potassium – that is to say, they make it work better. Dr. Jarvis agrees.

He writes: "I have come to the conclusion that potassium alone is not as effective in producing results as potassium with associated minerals, some of which must activate the potassium.

"One reason for the versatility of apple cider vinegar as a remedy in Vermont folk medicine is that it associates minerals with potassium. These are phosphorus, chlorine, sodium, magnesium, calcium, sulfur, iron, fluorine, silicon and trace minerals."

The second reason vinegar makes potassium so effective is that it presents the mineral in an acid medium, "and nature always combines potassium with an acid. I'd have to guess potassium needs an acid medium to work," Blodgett concluded.

Proper Growth

"**D**rink your vinegar and you'll grow up big and strong" is probably not something you heard in your house when you were a child, but it would have been absolutely true had your mother said it.

Potassium's main function is to promote cell, tissue and organism growth. This also means that potassium is necessary to replace worn-out tissue and dead cells. Basically, it sustains life. Slow growth in a child – or a failure to grow – could well be a sign of potassium deficiency, and so are signs of premature aging such as loss of hair, tooth decay or fingernails that are either brittle and tear, or soft and bend. That means that young and old alike need plenty of potassium.

"Potassium requirements are at a maximum when they are being used in infancy to build body tissues. But the requirements continue throughout life and there is no substitute for potassium," Jarvis writes.

And there is no better source of potassium than vinegar – particularly apple cider vinegar.

Signs of a Potassium Deficiency

1. Loss of mental alertness; difficulty with decision-making; lapses in memory
2. More frequent episodes of mental and muscle fatigue; loss of stamina and easy tiring
3. Sensitivity to cold and a propensity to cold hands and feet
4. Calluses on the bottom of the feet and growing corns
5. Constipation troubles
6. Susceptibility to sickness; frequent colds
7. Temporary losses of appetite with bouts of nausea and vomiting
8. Slow healing of cuts and bruises
9. Frequent and bothersome itches
10. Bothersome tooth decay
11. Pimples
12. Twitching of the eyelids or the corners of the mouth
13. Muscle cramps, especially in the legs, most often at night
14. Difficulty relaxing
15. Difficulty sleeping
16. Soreness in the joints; other symptoms of arthritis

If you detect more than five of these signs, you could be suffering from a potassium deficiency. While it may be advisable to see a physician, remember that as you grow older you need more potassium. Since this mineral is non-toxic, it's a good idea to increase your intake of it whether you see a doctor or not.

How to Increase Potassium Intake

1. Shake paprika in your food once or twice a day – it's a rich source of potassium.

2. Drink a glass of grape juice twice a day.

3. Alternatives are: a glass of apple juice or cranberry juice twice a day.

4. Eat a large banana every day.

5. Turn to grapefruits and other citrus as long as they're in season.

6. Eat two large potatoes each day (baked, boiled or cooked in some other way that does not bathe them in fat).

7. Eat two or three raw carrots a day.

8. Add tomatoes to your salad and tomato sauce to your pasta.

9. Eat at least two salads a day. Go heavy on the leafy greens, especially spinach, watercress, escarole, romaine lettuce and other dark leafy greens.

10. When cantaloupe is in season, make it a regular treat.

11. Snack on sunflower seeds.

Note: Dr. Earl Mindell, author of *The Vitamin Bible*, says alcohol, coffee, sugar and diuretics are the enemies of potassium. If you drink large amounts of coffee, you may ironically find yourself the victim of frequent fatigue. That is the direct result of potassium depletion.

Infection

Vinegar can help you fight off infection, as well. It does this by simply keeping fluids where they belong: in your body cells, not in bacteria.

Here's the way that works. Bacteria need moisture to thrive. They pull fluids out of your body's cells for their own purposes. If they multiply and your resistance is down, the process can go unchecked and you can become very sick. The end result of this process is death, naturally, but there are, fortunately, a number of medicines available today to prevent that.

The way to defeat bacterial infections, then, is to keep moisture in the cells and not let the germs get to it.

According to Dr. Jarvis: "If there is enough potassium in each body cell, it will draw moisture from the bacteria, instead of the bacteria taking moisture from the body cells.

"It is by taking care to eat foods which are a source of potassium, such as fruit, berries, edible leaves, edible roots and honey, and by the use of apple cider vinegar that the body cells are provided with the moisture-attracting potassium needed to win the contest with bacteria."

In addition, Dr. Blodgett explained to me that many of the medicines used to combat bacterial illnesses work on the same principle: by depriving bacteria of moisture and thus keeping fluids inside the cells.

Healthy Digestion

Good digestion means good health. Two teaspoons of apple cider vinegar to a glass of water at each meal is helpful in maintaining the health of your digestive tract, and in turn, the all-around health of your body.

Apple cider vinegar destroys microorganisms, including bacteria, fungi, viruses and others, and prevents poisons from reaching the rest of your system.

This effect is so potent that it can even protect you from

Continued on Pg. 42

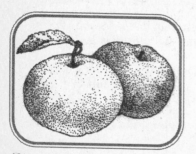

Strong Circulation

As long as you can keep your circulation system free from obstructions and keep your blood flowing freely, you dramatically reduce your risk of suffering a heart attack. The slow accumulation of fat and plaque deposits inside the blood vessels eventually chokes off the blood supply and hardens veins and arteries that need to be strong yet supple.

The major culprit for this process is our usually out-of-balance diet.

But apple cider vinegar can help.

"There is very little doubt that one of the functions of potassium is to keep the tissue soft and pliable," Dr. Jarvis wrote. "Potassium is to the soft tissues what calcium is to the hard tissues (bones) of the body. There is little doubt that potassium slows up the hardening processes that menace the whole blood vessel system."

One of the side benefits tied to improved circulation is clearer thinking. Mental activity is more effective because more oxygen reaches the brain. One of potassium's many benefits is that it promotes oxygenation of the blood.

food poisoning if you accidentally eat some fish, meat or other food that has spoiled slightly. Of course, it is always better to eat good, fresh food and avoid the problem in the first place. But it is helpful to know that you can avoid discomfort if you are accidentally sidelined.

This is especially useful information for the summer picnic season, which is also prime time for food poisoning. Unsuspecting vacationers can end a day of swimming, tennis and horseshoes writhing in agony from diarrhea and the rest of these wickedly upsetting digestive crises.

During the warm months, people who like to enjoy the outdoors also bring along lots of food – which they leave standing unrefrigerated, thus giving bacteria a wonderful opportunity to firmly take charge. The apple cider vinegar treatment can make the difference between health and illness.

And if you accidentally eat contaminated food, a teaspoon of apple cider vinegar added to a glass of water can treat the illness when most people assume it's too late – when symptoms are present.

"When there is food poisoning with vomiting, if you should attempt to drink a whole glass at once, the stomach will not accept it. But a small amount every few minutes can be kept down," recommends Jarvis.

"An ordinary drinking glass will hold about 50 teaspoons, and teaspoonful doses will require about four hours. When the contents of the first glass have been taken, another should be prepared in the same way and the dose increased to two or more teaspoons every five minutes. This will add another two hours of treatment. A third glassful should be prepared and taken one small swallow every 15 minutes."

If you wake up with nausea and vomiting or other symptoms of digestive upsets, he advises following the apple cider vinegar and water treatment throughout the day. By suppertime, you should be able to eat something light and easily digestible. Be sure to take extra vinegar and water five times a day or more for the next three days.

Kidney
and
Bladder

Apple cider vinegar has another important use as well. It keeps the kidneys and bladder doing their vital work of eliminating waste from the body.

It combats inflammation of the kidneys, which can lead to a back-up of toxins and eventually to blood poisoning. The acid nature of vinegar makes the environment in the urinary tract unpleasant for germs. Two teaspoons of vinegar in water will even quiet a potentially dangerous condition called *pyelitis*, in which pus cells originating in the bladder are present in the urine.

Fight Fat & Other Helpful Hints

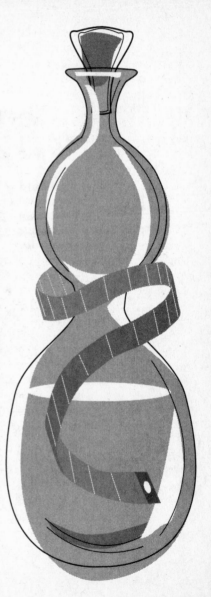

Everybody's looking for the magic bullet that will allow them to eat steak and subs and french fries with ice cream for dessert and still stay skinny.

I'm afraid I have to let you know that apple cider vinegar is not this kind of magic bullet.

But it can do something very important for you in your drive to get slim – or stay slim. Apple cider vinegar can help kick that metabolism of yours into high gear. And that means that your body is more likely to burn fat than to store it as unsightly flab. So there's a lot of good news for you here. Once again, you have the potassium content to thank for this, because it is potassium that promotes the proper chemical reactions in your body. And the acid nature of the vinegar makes certain that the conditions your body requires for fat burning are just right.

Do I hear you say that you're not sure if you're overweight or not? These days we have all kinds of means to determine this. We have digital scales, insurance company weight tables linked to height, and so on and so on. It's all around us. Dr. Jarvis looked at it from a rather more old-fashioned, homespun perspective.

"If the waist measurement is greater than that of the chest, or the chin is inclined to be double, then it is generally safe to conclude that the normal physiology and biochemistry in the body are disturbed." Read: You're too fat if it takes more tape to measure around your waist or hips than your chest.

"When this happens, Vermont folk medicine depends on apple cider vinegar to bring about a disappearance of fat."

The good news is that you don't have to make any frightening, major alterations in your daily diet. Just make sure, honestly, that you take care to avoid those foods that your experience has shown absolutely pack on the pounds around your waistline or your hips. For most people, sweets, chips, other snacks and burgers are likely to be the prime culprits. I know they are from my own experience. But don't ever let me hear you say that it is bread, potatoes or pasta that make you fat, because they really do not.

Fat is fattening, and starchy foods simply do not contain any fat. Meats, whole milk and cheese, pastries, snacks and junk food are the prime sources of fat. And so it is always the butter, sour cream or cheese that you add to starchy foods that actually put on the weight. It definitely is not the bread, spaghetti or potatoes.

What seems like less-than-wonderful news is that vinegar cannot help you lose 10 pounds in 10 days. The actual weight loss will be a good deal more gradual.

But in fact, that is really good news because researchers have shown over and over that it's weight that's lost gradually that, in the long-run, stays off.

Easy Slimming

As the good doctor says: "If a woman between five feet and five feet six inches tall weighing 210 pounds...takes two teaspoons of apple cider vinegar in a glass of water at each meal, she will weigh about 180 pounds at the end of two years. If a man has a paunch, he will lose the paunch in two years' time."

Since the vinegar will help you burn fat instead of store it, your daily activities will help you shed inches (and rolls) much more quickly than pounds.

Says Dr. Blodgett: "If a woman whose dress fits tightly will sip two teaspoons of apple cider vinegar in a glass of water at each meal, she will find at the end of two months that she can take her dress in one inch at the waistline. At the end of two more months, she will be able to take it in another inch and, by the end of the fifth month, one more inch.

"At the end of one year of taking apple cider vinegar in this amount, a woman who wears a size 50 dress will fit into a size 42, and one who wears a size 20, a size 18. Also, a woman who wears a size 16 will fit into a size 14."

Dr. Blodgett called the weight-loss plan completely simple and incredibly effective. It certainly sounds easy.

Sleep Deficit

Chronic fatigue is like an alarm clock waking you from a sound sleep. It alerts you that a dramatic change must take place quickly. This is a fancy way of saying that fatigue is a warning sign of impending illness.

A recent study at Cornell University showed that more than 50 million Americans suffer from sleep deficit and the resulting fatigue. Translation: They don't sleep enough. The solution, of course, is to get more shut-eye. But how?

Most of us are yawning and dragging around with heavy eyelids most of the time because there is so much to do in this get-up-and-go society of ours. When Dr. Blodgett would see the circles under my eyes, he would point out to me that I should go to bed ear-

Continued on Pg. 48

FOLK REMEDY

"To cope with chronic fatigue," Jarvis reports, "Vermont folk medicine knows no better treatment than this: Add three teaspoonsful of apple cider vinegar to a cup of honey, placing the mixture in a wide-mouthed bottle or jar that will admit a teaspoon. Keep the jar in a bedroom. Take two teaspoonsful of the mixture when preparing for bed."

Blodgett explains that this simple method should put you to sleep within half an hour. If you're still staring at the ceiling, take two more teaspoonsful and another at any time you wake up and feel you can't get back to sleep.

"This is far superior to the usual 'lullaby pills', because it is a treatment based on nature's own infallible knowledge of bodily requirements: Being harmless, it can be taken indefinitely. The honey may be taken by itself to produce sleep, but combining it with the apple cider vinegar is more effective."

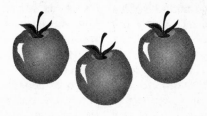

lier. He would add that artificial lighting is a relatively new invention, and that in the days before Thomas Edison, people used to go to bed not long after sunset and wake with the sunrise. Obviously times have changed and that is no longer possible or practical. But most of us could do with one more hour of sleep a night.

Above all, you want to stay away from sedatives, sleeping pills, narcotics or alcohol to help you. Once again, it's apple cider vinegar to the rescue.

Another way to overcome fatigue is to use apple cider vinegar in your bath. Add a half-pint to a tub full of bath water and immerse yourself in it for 15 minutes. The skin will absorb some of the vinegar, and the potassium in it, and pep you up. One note: Use the vinegar in the bath water instead of soap. It will clean your skin quite effectively. Yet another way to perk yourself up is to add several ounces to a sinkful of water. Splash it on your shoulders, arms, in

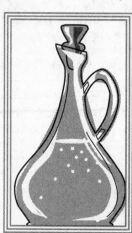

your armpits, on your chest, stomach, neck and face. Don't dry it with a towel, but let it soak in. You will find it quite refreshing.

For migraines, stress or headaches – apple cider vinegar is worth a try.

Many naturopathic physicians believe that most headaches have a single cause: too much alkaline in the system. When the body chemistry is changed back to a natural acidity, headaches usually disappear or become mild and more manageable.

Dr. Jarvis explains that you can restore that level of natural acidity by taking apple cider vinegar in water in the morning and evening and at every meal. If your headaches are bad, try doubling the amount of vinegar. He also recommends two teaspoonsful of honey at each meal to prevent a headache.

"If the headache has appeared, however, take a tablespoon of honey at once. Since it requires no process of digestion and will quickly be in the bloodstream, the headache will often begin to lessen by the end of a half-hour. If not, another teaspoonful of honey should be taken."

A vinegar vapor is also effective in relieving migraines. Put equal parts apple cider vinegar and water in a pan on the stove and bring it to a slow boil. Lean your head over and inhale as the fumes begin to rise from the basin.

Says Jarvis: "Inhale fumes for 75 breaths. Generally you will find that the headache stops for about half an hour. If it starts again, it will be about 50 percent less severe. The use of headache tablets can be stopped if the apple cider vinegar fumes method is employed."

Blood Pressure

Modern research bears out the folklore. A diet high in protein – because most of our protein comes from meat, it's generally also high in fat – and low in carbohydrates is a major contributor to elevated blood pressure. Every major health organization in the country agrees with that assessment, recom-mending a low-fat, high-fiber diet (carbohydrates are the best sources of fiber) to combat the condi-tion. This step will also pre-vent the likelihood of heart attacks and strokes that re-sult from hypertension.

A high-protein/high-fat diet turns the blood alkaline, which thickens it. That's one of the primary contributing factors to high blood pressure. Apple cider vinegar converts the blood acidity, thins it, lowers the blood pressure and makes circulation less of a strain.

Here is Jarvis's plan to lower high blood pressure:

1. Increase the daily intake of acid in organic form, either as apple cider vinegar, apples, grapes, cranberries or their juices.

2. Change to a more bal-anced diet. Ask the American Heart Association, the Ameri-can Cancer Society or a local dietitian for guidelines to a heart-healthy diet that's low in fat and high in fiber. It will automatically give you an ad-vantage in the war on high blood pressure.

3. Change from wheat prod-ucts (breads, muffins, cereals) to corn, oats, rye or rice. They will assist the shift from alkalinity to acidity within you and reduce strain on your kidneys – kidney damage and eventual failure is an often-overlooked complication of high blood pressure.

4. Give up salt and salty foods. This will reverse the blood's tendency to retain so much fluid – a prime cause of hypertension.

An apple cider vinegar gargle brings marked relief to sore throats. Use one teaspoonful to a glass of water and gargle with a mouthful of the solution every hour. Then swallow the solution, so it reaches the lower parts of the throat you can't touch by gargling. Repeat with a second mouthful. As pain lessens, increase intervals between gargling to every two hours.

The gargling kills strep germs, Jarvis reports. "Much to my surprise, I learned that this treatment could cure a streptococcic sore throat in 24 hours. As a rule, the patient became free of symptoms even before the Vermont state laboratory confirmed that the culture showed the presence of streptococci."

By the way, the apple cider vinegar treatment can also eliminate uncomfortable and embarrassing postnasal drip. This is caused by a production of excess mucus, which seeps out of the sinus cavities into the throat. It seems like a mere annoyance, but it is a perfect breeding ground for bacteria and other germs. If you suffer from this seemingly minor condition, it places you at more or less constant risk of throat and upper respiratory infection.

Apple cider vinegar, taken on a daily basis, can bring you arthritis relief by helping dissolve calcium deposits in joints and whisking them away for excretion.

As the blood becomes alkaline and thick, the solid particles in it precipitate out, and drop where they may in the body. For example, fat and cholesterol particles, blood clots, calcium and other materials filter out of the bloodstream to form hard and deadly atherosclerotic plaque on the inside walls of the arteries. In the same way, calcium may form deposits inside joints, making movement difficult and painful, and causing inflammation.

Jarvis, quoting folk healers in his native New England and backing them up from his own research, believes that by taking apple cider vinegar and water every day, you lower your blood's natural alkalinity, bringing it closer to an acid state.

Best of All, It's 'Green'

The long list of chemicals and additives you will find in most detergents and cleansers today may well be hazardous to your health. They are certainly dangerous to any child who wanders into a cupboard filled with drain cleaner, spot remover or floor wax – and drinks some or splashes some in the eyes. And once you throw the dregs down the drain or toss the packaging in the garage (which means years in a landfill), these chemicals and materials harm the earth.

Luckily, there are environmentally safe products for housework and they are just as effective as anything you can buy – in most cases, a lot cheaper. In fact, you probably have many of them in your kitchen already: baking soda, lemon juice, vegetable oil, borax and old-fashioned hot water.

At the head of the list put vinegar. Look at the many ways it can be used:

● **Air freshening:** Commercial air fresheners deaden nerves in your nose to diminish your sense of smell, not the odors. Set 2-4 Tbs of vinegar in open dishes.

● **Dishwashing liquid:** This is the number one cause of child poisoning among household products. And it's mostly made of non-biodegradeable detergents, with lots of chemical additives. Use liquid or powdered soap such as Ivory instead, adding 2-3 tsp of vinegar.

● **Drain cleaners:** Usually containing lye, hydrochloric and sulfuric acids, they're lethal. Once a week, plug the overflow drain with a wet rag, pour ¼ cup baking soda down the drain, followed by ½ cup vinegar. Close the drain until the fizzing stops. Flush with one gallon boiling water.

● **Floor cleaners:** One-half cup of vinegar (white, preferably) mixed in ½ gallon of warm water cuts through dull, greasy film on no-wax linoleum.

● **Furniture polishes:** Many wood polishes contain phenol, which caused cancer during laboratory tests on rats. Mix vegetable or lemon oil and vinegar in equal parts and apply as a thin coat. Rub in well.

● **Glass cleaners:** Commercial products contain ammonia, which is a poison. Try this instead: Use alcohol first to clean off the residue of other cleaners, then clean glass with a mixture of white vinegar and warm water in equal proportions.

● **Metal polishes:** For aluminum, soak overnight in a mixture of vinegar and water, then rub. For brass, mix equal parts of salt and flour with a little vinegar, then rub. For chrome, rub with undiluted vinegar. For copper, rub with a paste of vinegar, salt and flour, or hot vinegar and salt.

● **Mold and mildew:** Make a concentrated solution of borax or vinegar and water to clean the affected areas. When you're sure it's mildew, try a mixture of vinegar and salt first.

● **Toilet cleaners:** Blueing agents contain chlorine and hydrochloric acid, which can burn your eyes and skin. Use soap and borax to remove stubborn rings, and white vinegar for lime buildup. Or sprinkle baking soda into the bowl, drizzle the vinegar and scour.

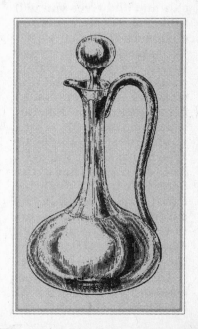

Making Vinegar at Home

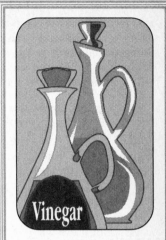

You can easily make your own apple cider vinegar or blackberry vinegar. In addition, you can also add tasty herbs to commercially prepared vinegars purchased in any supermarket.

In her book *Herbal Medicine*, Dr. Dian Dincin Buchman, Ph.D., of the State University of New York at Purchase and at the College of New Rochelle, who is one of the world's most noted writers and lecturers on the benefits of natural medicine, enthuses about the benefits of vinegars.

She recommends this invigorating drink, which relieves fatigue and also helps to dissolve arthritic and gouty deposits:

Combine 1 Tbs of uncooked honey and 1 Tbs of a good apple cider vinegar. Add this mixture to a glass of water. You may

Vinegar: 1. a sour liquid used as a condiment or preservative that is obtained by acetic fermentation of dilute alcoholic liquids (as fermented cider, malt beer or wine) or of dilute distilled alcohol and is often seasoned, esp. with herbs **2.** disagreeableness of speech, disposition or attitude **3.** a pharmaceutical solution of the active principles of drugs in dilute acetic acid usually prepared by maceration
– Webster's Dictionary

use a little less honey if you are making a pitcherful. This excellent drink is good for small children (although not for newborn infants), and this ancient combination of sweet and sour

53

plus water normalizes the body.

She writes: "Apple cider vinegar is useful externally to alleviate pain and help reduce sprains. I use at least a cup at a time in the bath to alleviate muscle soreness. I also splash it directly on my shoulders, arms, chest and torso to restore flagging energy. I don't really know why apple cider vinegar patted on the body or placed in the bathwater will overcome body fatigue, but it does.

"Diluted apple cider vinegar may be used in small amounts to help reduce fever and may also be splashed or sponged on the patient to reduce the temperature. Carefully sponge the body in sections and friction dry, and do not allow the rest of the body to be in a draft."

Herb vinegars are also excellent when used to cleanse sickrooms and wash the patient during any bacterial illness or during an epidemic of any kind.

Doing It Yourself

You will need a wide-mouthed jar or crock, a cover for the crock, and the peelings, cores and bruised apples left after making applesauce or apple pie, writes Dr. Buchman. Place the leftover pieces of apple in the crock, and cover with cold water. Place the lid on the crock, and store it in a warm place.

Occasionally lift the cover and add whatever additional peels, cores and apple pieces you can. Strain off the froth as you go along. When the vinegar smells and tastes right, strain out the apple pieces. Pour the vinegar into sterilized bottles and cork for further use.

Aeration is the key to souring a vinegar. If you wish to quicken the fermentation process, add a small amount of live yeast in a brown paper bag to your crock or keg.

To aerate as farmers once did, keep two barrels with spigots. In one barrel, make the vinegar as described above. In the second barrel, keep matchstick-thin sticks of birch or beech boards. After a few days, open the faucet and allow the cider to dribble through the birch or beech boards.

As soon as the second barrel fills up, pour the vinegar into the first barrel again. This process may be repeated several times.

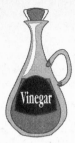
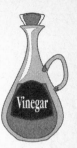

Special Vinegars

Here are some of Dr. Buchman's favorite vinegar recipes:

Blackberry Vinegar

4 pounds fresh blackberries
Enough malt vinegar to cover blackberries
1 pound sugar for every pint
extracted blackberry juice
Note: Sugar can be replaced with glycerine.
See the recipe for 'Blackberry Glycerite'.

Wash the blackberries in cold running water. Place in a glass, earthenware or ceramic pot. Cover with malt vinegar for three days. Stir once a day. Strain through a sieve and drain thoroughly by placing a plate on top and putting a weight on the plate. Let it drip all day. Measure the juice and allow one pound of sugar per pint of juice (for external use, glycerine is preferred – see next recipe). Simmer in another glass, ceramic or earthenware pot for five minutes. Collect and discard the top scum. Let cool, then bottle, cork and label.

Dr. Buchman reports that this vinegar is excellent for fevers, arthritis and gout. The dosage here is 1 Tbs dissolved in a large cup of distilled water. Use three times a day. This preparation will somewhat ease the pain and is said to eventually help dissolve arthritic deposits. This vinegar is also good for anemia and has helped many heart patients.

Modern Anti-Epidemic
Vinegar

1 quart apple cider vinegar
1 pound garlic buds for 8 oz juice
8 oz comfrey root
4 oz oak bark
4 oz marshmallow root
4 oz mullein flowers
4 oz rosemary flowers
4 oz lavender flowers
4 oz wormwood
4 oz black walnut leaves
12 oz glycerine

Make separate teas of each of the herbs. First soak each ounce of herb in clean spring water. After about half a day, simmer each herb separately for 10 minutes. Steep for half an hour. Strain out, simmer again, and reduce each herb so that it is concentrated. Press garlic buds into 8 oz of concentrated juice. Add 12 oz of glycerine to preserve it. Place in a large bottle. Label. Close. You may want to add paraffin for additional preservation power.

Dosage: 1-3 tsp during epidemics, or 1 tsp per hour if someone in the family is ill with a communicable disease. Dilute with water if too strong to the taste, or add to hot herbal tea.

Herb Vinegars for Face, Bath or Salad

Here are three more excellent herb vinegar recipes. You can use them as a refreshing, aromatic addition to bathwater or as an invigorating facial splash. They also make delightful dressings for salad.

1 qt apple cider vinegar
4 Tbs dried herbs (or 2 Tbs fresh herbs)

Place vinegar in a ceramic or glass pot. Bring to a brief boil. Turn off heat. Add herbs. Pour into vinegar jar. Use leftover vinegar for body wash or addition to bath.

1 qt apple cider vinegar
1 handful fresh mint or tarragon (or 3 Tbs dried mint)

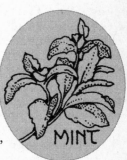

Wash mint, bruise leaves well and pack into jar. Cover tightly and let stand two weeks. Strain out the herbs. (If dried mint is used, first simmer the vinegar, bring to a boil, and then pour over the mint.)

½ pint apple cider vinegar
1 oz rose petals
¼ pint rosewater
½ pint vinegar (apple cider or white)
1 oz several different kinds of aromatic flowers
(examples: lavender, sweet violet, rosemary)

Mix and steep for two weeks.

Blackberry Glycerite

This recipe is almost the same as that for blackberry vinegar, but you use glycerine instead of the sugar. For every pint of the extracted juice, use 8 oz (½ pint) of glycerine. Simmer the blackberry vinegar and glycerine together for five minutes. Skim. Cool and place in a sterilized, labeled bottle. Store in a cool place.

This glycerite of blackberry can be used in the same way as the vinegar. For painful joints, heat this preparation in small quantities. Dip in a folded cloth. Apply hot cloth to painful joints several times a day.

Four Thieves

Vinegar of the Four Thieves is one of the most interesting legends in the fascinating history of herbalism, reports Dr. Buchman. She says the recipe may actually have been devised by an apothecary, Richard Forthave, and that the success and usefulness of the remedy created its own myth. This recipe has been in use for centuries, but legend has it that it was discovered during a devastating bubonic plague.

Four thieves who had safely ransacked empty plague-ridden houses were caught by policemen and brought before the French judges in Marseilles.

The judges wondered aloud how these thieves had resisted the plague, especially since they were in and out of plague-infested homes.

"We drink and wash with this vinegar preparation every few hours," they answered.

In return for giving the recipe, the thieves were given their freedom.

There are several Four Thieves vinegars. Dr. Buchman received the simplest recipe from the notebook of a Virginia housewife.

She combined a handful of each of the anti-disease herbs and steeped them in apple cider vinegar. After the initial two-week steeping, she added garlic buds.

This aromatic and antibacterial vinegar is an excellent wash for floors, walls, sinks, bedsteads, pots and pans in sickrooms, bathrooms and kitchens. It will offset a damp-weather smell in a house and be a helpful floor and wall wash in a room overcrowded with people.

Externally, this vinegar may be used in small proportions in a bath or diluted for body wash. You can use ordinary apple cider vinegar in an undiluted state if desired, but some of the herbs in this recipe are too strong for the skin, and the vinegar must be diluted.

Internally, the safest, most effective dose is a teaspoon at a time in water – and no more than 1 Tbs an hour (Remember: 3 tsp equals 1 Tbs). This acts as a strong general preventive medicine.

Vinegar of the Four Thieves

2 qts apple cider vinegar
2 Tbs lavender
2 Tbs rosemary
2 Tbs sage
2 Tbs wormwood
2 Tbs rue
2 Tbs mint
2 Tbs garlic buds

Combine the dried herbs (except the garlic), and steep in the vinegar in the sun for two weeks. Strain and rebottle. Label. Add several cloves of garlic. Close lid. When garlic has steeped for several days, strain out. Melt paraffin wax around the lid to preserve the contents, or add 4 oz of glycerine for preservation.

Note dosage above.

SAGE

Great
Garlic
Recipes

The most wondrous substances nature has to offer come in the form of wholesome food. They don't need any magical healing properties beyond the nourishment and sustenance they supply – fiber, vitamins, minerals and other elements. They are the stuff of life, and there's little else you require for health, happiness and a long and productive time on earth.

Plant foods are the best friends you have, and Mother Nature intended you to eat them in huge quantities every day. If you're eating a food, and it came out of the ground as a root, stalk, stem or leaf, it is almost certainly high in fiber, free of dangerous, artery-clogging fats and cholesterol, extremely low in calories and loaded with goodness. This is also true for whole-grain foods such as rice, oats, corn, rye, millet, etc.

Health agencies, researchers, the National Academy of Sciences – your family doctor – all recommend a diet that is high in fiber. A diet in which the calories come from 60 percent carbohydrates, 10 percent protein and no more than 30 percent fat, can protect you from serious illnesses such as cancer, heart disease and diabetes.

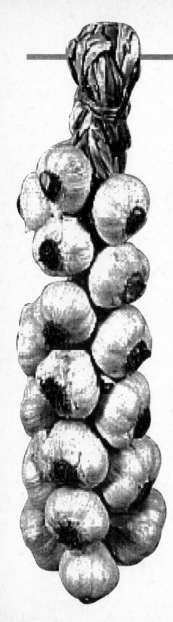

Other experts recommend even less fat – as little as 20 or in some cases 10 percent of total calories from fat.

You may wonder what all that means.

You can place yourself in the ballpark and not have to worry or count or calculate precisely if you follow a few simple steps. First, eat cereal with some oat bran sprinkled on it for breakfast, with a piece of fruit and some toast or a roll. Eat two salads a day, one at lunch and the other at dinner. Consume at least three cups of raw vegetables a day; plan one meatless meal every week; and limit the amount of meat you eat to four ounces a day.

This will enable you to eat more than ever before, and weigh less! This is the way that nature, and your body, intended you to eat. This is the natural way.

Bearing that in mind, here are some wondrous recipes. In *The Book of Garlic*, Lloyd J. Harris says, "There are a number of recipes that treat garlic as it should be treated – as a vegetable and not merely a spice, herb, seasoning or flavoring." He suggests a number of creative ways to bake, boil, sauté and broil garlic. The results are delicious, particularly since cooking mellows the bulb.

Here are some mouth-watering recipes for garlic lovers

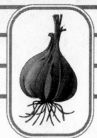

Halved Heads
of Garlic in Sauce

4 heads garlic
1 Tbs olive oil
2 Tbs butter
1 cup chicken stock
1 cup white wine
Pinch of thyme
Salt and pepper

Cut each head of garlic in half.

Heat the oil and butter in a saucepan over moderate heat. Sauté the bulbs, cut side down, until the garlic meat begins to brown.

Add the chicken stock, wine and herbs.

Cover the pan with a tight lid, and braise over low heat until the liquid is reduced and thickened and the garlic cloves are soft when poked with a knife.

Serve cut side up on the plate and spoon some of the stock over each half.

Eat the garlic like an artichoke, using your teeth and lips to pull the purée out of the skins.

The sauce is also delicious spooned over chicken.

Roasted Garlic

Preheat oven to 350°

10-12 large garlic cloves, peeled
2 Tbs butter
1 Tbs peanut oil
1 Tbs olive oil
Salt to taste
Pinch of white pepper

Heat the butter, peanut oil and olive oil in a casserole over medium heat. Add peeled cloves, side by side, and make sure they are well coated. Bake for 20 minutes, basting from time to time. Add salt and pepper.

Serve as an appetizer with toast or as a vegetable side dish.

Charcoal Roasted
Whole Garlic

This variation on the recipe above
is a Middle Eastern specialty.

Place whole bulbs of garlic, basted with oil, salt and pepper, directly in white hot but not flaming coals. When they're lightly browned, they're ready. Allow the bulbs to cool and break off the cloves.

Parsley Salad
with Garlic Dressing

3 large bunches
parsley

5 cloves garlic,
crushed

¼ cup salad oil

Juice of large lemon

1 tsp salt

½ tsp pepper

1 lb mushrooms,
sliced

4 Tbs grated
Parmesan

Rinse parsley thoroughly. Remove stems and separate into small clusters. Toss parsley and Parmesan. Add mushrooms and refrigerate until ready to serve.

Combine garlic, oil, lemon juice, salt and pepper. Mix thoroughly. Pour over salad right before serving.

The parsley neutralizes garlic breath.

Garlic Purée

2 dozen or more garlic cloves

1 Tbs olive oil

Salt and pepper

Herbs of your choice

Place whole, unpeeled cloves in a pot of boiling water for about 20 minutes or until clove meat is very soft. Drain and cool.

When cool, remove skins and place cloves in a food processor or blender. Purée, adding salt, pepper, herbs and olive oil. Pour into a glass jar and refrigerate.

Use to thicken and flavor sauces, soups, stews, dressings and dips. Spread on croutons and serve with soups and salads or use as a sandwich spread for leftovers. Serve over hot rice.

Poached Garlic
with Butter

Place peeled or unpeeled cloves in gently boiling water. Simmer until soft, testing with a fork. Strain. Put garlic and about 1 Tbs butter per five cloves into a warm pan. Serve simply with the melted butter or sauté until lightly browned. Add salt and pepper to taste.

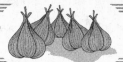

Garlic Soup

12 servings

3 Tbs olive oil

30 large garlic cloves, chopped

2 cans chicken broth or 1 qt homemade

2 cups water

1 tsp salt

1 tsp pepper

2 bay leaves

1 fresh jalapeno pepper, seeded and chopped

1 cup half-and-half

12 slices French bread

Parmesan cheese, grated

In saucepan, heat oil on medium. Add garlic and sauté until soft and golden. Add chicken broth, water, salt, pepper, bay leaves and jalapeno pepper. Simmer 5 minutes.

Pour into blender and purée. Return to saucepan. Stir in half-and-half and heat through.

Toast bread lightly. Sprinkle with Parmesan cheese and broil 3 minutes or until cheese is golden and bubbly.

Stuffed Chicken Wings

1 medium head
garlic, chopped

½ lb smoked turkey

12 chicken wings

Tempura batter
(any brand will do)

1 qt cooking oil

Combine garlic and turkey. Set aside.

Remove large bone in chicken wing, being careful not to cut the outer skin. Stuff cavity with meat and garlic. Dip stuffed wings in tempura batter. Fry in very hot oil. Cook until golden brown. Drain on paper towels. Serve hot.

Hot and Garlicky Wings

Preheat oven to 375°

2 lbs chicken wings

3 heads fresh garlic

1 cup plus 1 Tbs
olive oil

10-15 drops Tabasco
sauce

1 cup Parmesan
cheese, grated

1 cup Italian-style
bread crumbs

1 tsp black pepper

Disjoint chicken wings, discarding tips. Rinse and pat dry. Set aside.

Separate garlic into cloves and peel. Place garlic, olive oil and Tabasco in blender or food processor and purée.

Combine Parmesan, bread crumbs and pepper.

Dip wings in the garlic purée and roll in bread crumb mixture, one at a time, coating thoroughly.

Coat a shallow nonstick baking pan with oil and add wings in a single layer. Drizzle with remaining garlic purée and sprinkle with any remaining crumb mixture.

Bake for 45 to 60 minutes until brown and crisp.

Eggplant Antipasto

Preheat oven to 350°

4-6 eggplants
(Chinese or
Japanese)

4 tomatoes, chopped

1 head of garlic,
crushed or finely
chopped

Fresh basil, finely
chopped or dried

Salt and pepper
to taste

Parmesan cheese,
grated (optional)

Olive oil

Cut eggplant in half, lengthwise, then again crosswise so you end up with 4 pieces. Make several deep slits into the meat of the eggplant without cutting through to the skin. Stuff chopped tomatoes into the slits, place garlic on top and sprinkle with basil and salt and pepper to taste. Sprinkle with Parmesan cheese, if so desired. Drizzle with lots of olive oil. Bake for 25-30 minutes.

Gilroy Chili

3 cloves garlic, minced

2 large onions,
finely chopped

2 Tbs olive oil

2 lbs lean ground beef

1 8-oz can stewed
tomatoes

1 4-oz can green chilies

2 cups beef stock

1 Tbs chili powder

1 Tbs ground cumin

1 tsp salt

¼ tsp pepper

In a large skillet, slowly brown the garlic and onions in olive oil; stir and cook until tender. Raise heat, add meat and cook until done. Add all other ingredients. Cover and reduce heat. Cook about 45 minutes more.

Patrician Escargots

4 servings
Preheat oven to 350°

4 heads garlic
½ cup olive oil
½ cup butter
1 small onion,
  finely chopped
1 tsp fresh rosemary,
  finely chopped
¼ tsp ground thyme
2 dashes nutmeg

Salt and pepper
  to taste
24 large canned snails
½ cup parsley,
  chopped
24 medium to large
  fresh mushrooms
12 pieces thin-sliced
  white bread

Peel garlic and chop into fine pieces. Place olive oil and butter in a frying pan over medium heat. When butter is melted, add onion, garlic, rosemary and thyme. Then add nutmeg, salt and pepper. Reduce heat to low and add snails and parsley; simmer for 30 minutes.

While snails are simmering, clean and remove stems from mushrooms. Arrange mushroom caps upside down in a 2-inch-deep baking dish and place one snail into each mushroom cap. Pour garlic mixture over snails, cover with foil and bake for 30 minutes.

While snails are baking, remove the crusts from the bread slices and cut each slice into 4 squares. Toast bread. Serve with escargots.

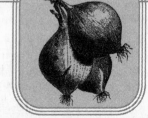

Ambrosial Grape Leaves

10 servings
Preheat oven to 350°

1 jar grape leaves

1 onion, chopped

2 Tbs butter or olive oil

1½ lbs ground lamb

1-2 heads garlic, peeled and chopped

Salt and pepper

6-8 oz pine nuts (pignoli)

2 cups seedless raisins

2-3 Tbs sugar

6 Tbs cinnamon

1 stick (8 oz) butter, melted

Rinse grape leaves, cut off stems and lay flat.

Sauté onion in butter or olive oil until translucent. Add lamb, crumbling as it cooks. When no longer pink, stir in garlic and season with salt and pepper to taste.

Remove from heat and add pine nuts, raisins, sugar and cinnamon.

Place 2-3 Tbs of the mixture in the center of each grape leaf. Fold the leaf over the filling and roll up like a cigar. Place the stuffed grape leaves in a single layer in a baking dish. Dribble with melted butter. Bake for 20 minutes and serve hot.

Garlic Plumped Chicken

4 servings
Preheat oven to 400°

3 heads fresh garlic	¼ cup chicken stock
1 chicken (3½ to 4 lbs)	¼ cup marsala (or port or red wine)
¾ lb fresh mushrooms	¼ cup heavy cream
8 Tbs unsalted butter	Juices from cavity of roasted chicken
Salt and pepper	

Wrap garlic in foil and roast in preheated 400° oven about 30 minutes or until garlic is cooked and soft. Cool, then squeeze out pulp of cloves and set aside. Rinse chicken and pat dry. With breast side up, beginning at the neck end, separate the skin from flesh, loosening as far into the legs and wings as possible without tearing skin. This creates a pocket for the stuffing. Set chicken aside.

Clean mushrooms and finely chop. Sauté in 2 Tbs butter over high heat until all moisture has evaporated, stirring and taking care not to burn. Cool. Combine ⅔ garlic pulp, mushrooms and remaining 6 Tbs butter. Mix thoroughly; add salt and pepper to taste. Stuff chicken with garlic mixture. Fill the pocket, spreading evenly with fingers.

Rub outside of chicken with a little butter and sprinkle with fresh ground pepper. Place chicken breast side up in a roasting pan with a rack and roast at 400° for approximately 1½ hours until juices in thigh run clear. Reserve juices from cavity; carefully cut up chicken into serving pieces and keep warm.

Combine remaining third of garlic pulp, reserved juices, stock, wine and cream in a small saucepan over high heat. Stir until thickened. Serve with chicken.

Linguine With
Caramelized Garlic

3-4 servings

3 heads fresh garlic
3 Tbs olive oil
1 Tbs chopped,
  fresh thyme
⅛ cup chicken stock
  (if using canned,
  use regular, not
  double strength)

Salt and pepper
  to taste
6 oz linguine
2 eggs, beaten
3 oz freshly grated
  Parmesan cheese

Separate garlic cloves. Immerse in boiling water for 30 seconds and peel. Heat oil in large sauté pan over medium-low heat. Add garlic. Reduce heat to low and very slowly sauté garlic until golden brown. Stir frequently. Be careful not to burn garlic. It will take approximately 20 minutes for the garlic to reach this state. Stir in fresh thyme. Cook 2 minutes longer. Add chicken stock, salt and pepper. Simmer 5 minutes.

Meanwhile, cook linguine according to package directions. Drain. Toss linguine with eggs. Add to sauté pan and toss with Parmesan cheese. Adjust seasonings. Serve immediately.

THYME

Homemade Italian Sausage

9 lbs Boston butt pork roast, boned
3 oz salt
3 Tbs black pepper
¼ cup fresh garlic, finely chopped
3 Tbs crushed red chili pepper
Casings – pork small intestines
Optional: 2 Tbs fennel and 1 Tbs oregano

Grind pork roast with a coarse grind sausage blade. Add salt, black pepper, garlic, chili peppers and the options desired. Knead this mixture thoroughly for at least 10 minutes. When mixed properly, the mixture will stick to your hand for 3 or 4 seconds when held upside down.

Wash the casings thoroughly in water, inside and out. Tie one end closed and then pack the ingredients inside the casing tightly, making sure to remove all air and filling the voids. Tie the other end closed.

About every 4 or 5 inches, pinch the filled casing together and double the end back through in a looping motion. This will divide your sausage into individual connected pieces.

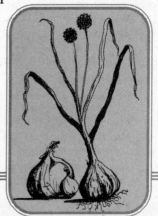

With a fork, prick each segment 3 or 4 times. Place the sausage in an uncovered container and refrigerate them for 3 days. This allows the ingredients to 'marry'. Sausage can also be dried or frozen.

Rainy Sunday Super Stuffed Shells

9 to 12 servings

2 Tbs olive oil
3 cloves garlic
¾ lb ground veal
¾ lb ground pork
1 10-oz package frozen chopped spinach
1 cup parsley, finely chopped
1 cup bread crumbs

2 eggs, beaten
3 cloves garlic, minced
3 Tbs Parmesan cheese, grated
Salt to taste
1 12-oz package jumbo pasta shells
3 cups tomato sauce

Mix ground veal and ground pork together. In a large skillet, heat the olive oil over medium heat and sauté three whole cloves of garlic until brown. Remove and discard garlic, add the veal and pork mixture and lightly brown. Drain excess fat and set aside to cool.

In a large mixing bowl, combine the cooked chopped spinach, parsley, bread crumbs, eggs, minced garlic and cheese. Blend well and salt to taste. Add cooled, browned meat and mix thoroughly.

Bring 3 quarts of salted water to a full boil. Carefully add the jumbo pasta shells. Cook the shells for 5 to 7 minutes. The shells should be undercooked for ease of handling. Drain and immediately rinse under plenty of cold water.

Preheat oven to 375°. Generously coat the bottom of an 8" x 11" baking dish with some of the tomato sauce. Using a teaspoon, fill the cooked shells with the stuffing and arrange decoratively in the baking dish. Spoon additional tomato sauce over each stuffed shell and cover the baking dish with aluminum foil. Bake for 35 to 45 minutes.

Nancy's Glorious Garlic Quiche

Pastry crust
(recipe follows)

3 heads fresh garlic,
separated and peeled

2 tsp Dijon-style
mustard

1 cup grated
Gruyere cheese

1 egg

¼ cup heavy cream

1 tsp nutmeg

¼ tsp pepper

Half fill a large saucepan with water. Add garlic cloves and bring to a boil. Drain garlic and repeat process with fresh water. Drain and reserve garlic. With back of spoon, smear mustard across bottom of pastry crust, which can be hot from oven or at room temperature. Distribute cheese evenly inside crust. In a food processor, purée reserved garlic with egg, cream, nutmeg and pepper for 30 seconds. Pour garlic mixture over cheese. Bake tart at 350° for 25 minutes, until filling is firm. Serve hot or at room temperature. Makes 8 servings.

Pastry Crust

1½ cups all-purpose
flour

1 tsp sugar

1 tsp salt

1 stick (8 oz) frozen
butter, cut into 6
pieces

¼ cup ice water

Preheat oven to 350°. In food processor, combine flour, sugar, salt and butter until mixture looks crumbly. With motor running, slowly add water. Mixture will gather in a ball. Wrap dough in plastic wrap and refrigerate for at least half an hour. Butter and flour inside of a 9-inch tart pan which has a removable bottom. Roll out dough to fit into pan. Trim edges. Line dough with foil and fill center with pie weights or dried beans. Bake for 20 minutes. Remove foil and weights. Continue baking crust for additional 10 minutes, until crust begins to brown.

Spaghettaccini Carolini

6 servings

1 lb spaghetti noodles

4 Tbs oil

¼ lb butter

24 cloves fresh garlic, peeled and chopped

1 lb fresh jumbo shrimp, peeled and butterflied

1 red bell pepper, thinly sliced

1 bunch broccoli, cut into serving size spears

2 cups fresh mushrooms

1 cup chopped fresh parsley

1 cup chopped green onions

1 Tbs dried red pepper

2 Tbs flour

½ cup dry white wine

1 pint heavy cream

1 small wedge (about 3 oz) Parmesan cheese, grated

Salt to taste

Cook noodles according to package directions in boiling water with 2 Tbs oil. Meanwhile, melt butter in large skillet over medium-high heat. Add chopped garlic and shrimp; cook until shrimp turns pink, but do not allow garlic to brown. Set aside. In another skillet, over medium-high heat, stir-fry red bell pepper and broccoli in remaining 2 Tbs oil. Cook until crisp-tender. Drain and set aside. Add mushrooms, half the parsley, onions and red pepper to garlic and shrimp; sauté for one minute. Add flour, mix thoroughly and add wine. Simmer for about 30 seconds, then add cream and heat thoroughly, stirring. Drain noodles and add to sauce with half the grated cheese. Toss gently until noodles are well-coated and cheese is melted. Salt lightly. If sauce is too thin, continue heating until sauce reduces to a creamy consistency. If sauce is too thick, add cream. Gently toss in the stir-fried vegetables. Garnish with remaining chopped parsley and grated cheese and serve immediately.

Scampi Alla 'Fireman Chef'

1 lb large prawns
8 sprigs fresh parsley
⅛ cup clarified butter
4 Tbs minced garlic
6 scallions, thinly sliced
Juice of a lemon (approximately 2 Tbs)
¼ cup dry white wine
Salt and freshly ground pepper to taste
Lemon slices for garnish

Shell and de-vein the prawns. Rinse and set aside. Reserve a few nice sprigs of parsley for garnish and mince the rest. Heat the clarified butter in a large sauté pan over medium heat. Lightly sauté the garlic for 1 to 2 minutes, being careful not to let it brown. Add the prawns, scallions, lemon juice and wine. Cook the mixture until the prawns turn pink and firm, a minute or two on each side. Be careful not to overcook.

At the last minute, add the minced parsley and season with salt and pepper. Serve the scampi on individual shells or small gratin dishes, garnished with a slice or two of lemon and a fresh parsley sprig.

Garlic Chicken Pineapple

4 servings

1 head fresh garlic, peeled

1 piece fresh ginger (1 inch square), peeled

5 Tbs vegetable oil

9 black peppercorns

5 cardamom pods

5 whole cloves

1 stick cinnamon

1 large onion (preferably red), chopped

1 chicken, skinned and cut up

2 potatoes, peeled and diced (optional)

1 can sliced pineapple, drained and cut in triangular pieces

In blender, grind garlic and ginger to form a smooth paste; add a little water for good consistency, but not too much. Heat oil and add peppercorns, cardamom, cloves, cinnamon and onion, cooking until light golden in color. Add garlic-ginger paste and cook about 5 minutes, stirring constantly. If this 'masala' is sticking to the pan, reduce heat to medium. Add chicken, cooking until browned, add about 1 cup water and deglaze pan. Reduce heat to medium-low, cover pan and let chicken cook 50 minutes or until tender. Add potatoes, if desired, after chicken has cooked 20 minutes. Just before serving, add pineapple.

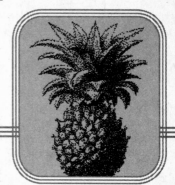

Gloria's Lamb Stew

This is lamb stew with a difference – chili peppers, garlic and fresh cilantro are the seasonings.

4 to 5 servings

1 cup fresh cilantro leaves (coriander)
1 whole head fresh garlic, peeled
2 or 3 fresh hot red or green peppers, seeded
⅓ cup olive oil
2 medium onions, finely chopped
4 lb lean boneless lamb, cut into 1-inch cubes
Salt and freshly ground pepper to taste
⅔ cup fresh orange juice
⅓ cup lime or lemon juice water
2 lb potatoes, peeled and sliced
1 lb fresh green peas, shelled or
2 pkg (10-oz each) frozen

In blender or food processor purée cilantro, garlic and peppers; set aside.

Heat oil in casserole or Dutch oven and sauté onions until soft. Stir in cilantro mixture and cook for a minute or two longer. Add lamb pieces and cook for about 5 minutes, turning to coat with sauce. Season to taste with salt and a generous amount of pepper. Add orange and lime or lemon juice and enough water to cover, about 1½ cups.

Cover and simmer until lamb is tender, about 1½ hours.

If desired, this dish may be refrigerated at this point in order to solidify and remove any excess fat. Let stand to bring to room temperature before heating. Boil potatoes and peas separately in salted water until tender. Drain and add to casserole. Bring casserole to a simmer and cook just long enough to heat through.

Garlic Pudding

During the First Garlic Festival, Digger Dan's, a Gilroy restaurant, featured this unusual dessert on their menu. Although the recipe calls for quite a lot of garlic, it is a light and flavorful dessert.

2 heads fresh garlic
1½ cups cold water
1 cup sugar
1 envelope unflavored gelatin
¼ cup lemon juice
1 tsp lemon peel, grated
2 egg whites
¼ tsp nutmeg
Custard sauce (recipe below)
¼ tsp salt

Wrap garlic heads in foil and bake until done (soft). Remove from foil and boil in water until flavor is transferred from bulbs to water and water is reduced to about 1¼ cups garlic water. In saucepan combine sugar, gelatin and salt. Add ½ cup garlic water; stir until dissolved and remove from heat. Add remaining ¾ cup garlic water, lemon juice and lemon peel. Chill until partially set. Turn into large bowl. Add egg whites and beat with electric mixer until mixture begins to hold its shape. Turn into mold. Chill until firm. Unmold and garnish with sprinkles of nutmeg and custard sauce.

Custard Sauce

4 egg yolks, beaten   2 cups milk
¼ cup sugar   Dash salt

In heavy saucepan, mix egg yolks with sugar, milk and salt. Cook over low heat until mixture coats spoon. Cool and serve over pudding.

Garlic Chip Cookies

Desserts made with garlic? Well, why not? Everyone who tasted them agreed they were delicious and would even be better with more garlic!

Makes 5 dozen cookies

10 cloves fresh garlic
Boiling water
½ cup maple syrup
1 cup butter, softened
¾ cup brown sugar
¾ cup sugar
2 eggs

1 tsp vanilla
½ tsp salt
2¼ cups chocolate chips
½ cup chopped nuts
2½ cups flour
1 tsp baking soda

Drop garlic cloves into boiling water for about 5 minutes until tender. Peel and chop garlic and soak in maple syrup for 20 minutes.

Meanwhile, cream butter, sugars, eggs and vanilla together until light and fluffy. Combine flour, baking soda and salt. Add to cream mixture. Then stir in chocolate chips and nuts.

Drain garlic and add to cookie batter. Blend well. Drop cookie batter by tablespoons onto ungreased cookie sheet about 2 inches apart. Bake at 375° for 8 to 10 minutes, until lightly browned. Remove from oven and cool on racks.

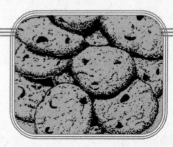

Garlic, Vinegar & Your Pets

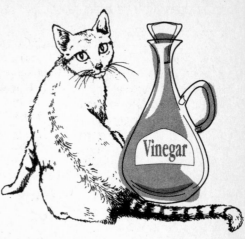

A California veterinarian calls it the 'poor man's penicillin'. It is an essential part of the daily diet of some of the world's most highly prized racehorses. You guessed it; it's lifesaving garlic – the natural way to keep your pets at their best.

Just listen to the animal experts sing its praises:

David Smith, DVM, of North Hills, CA, commonly prescribes garlic as part of his flea prevention program and for treating and preventing allergy flare-ups. He also believes it may help prevent certain cancers in pets.

Richard H. Pitcairn of Eugene, OR, author of *Natural Health for Dogs and Cats*, claims the tasty little bulbs help strengthen animals' digestion and intestinal tracts and eliminate worms. He also recom-

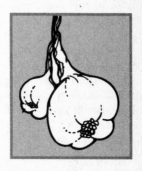

mends garlic for a pet that has been on a high meat or fish diet, that tends to put on weight or that suffers hip pain from arthritis or dysplasia.

Researchers at California's

81

Loma Linda University School of Medicine attribute garlic's ability to control parasites to its powerful antibacterial action. They say it controls the growth of microorganisms.

Veterinarian Gloria Dodd, who calls garlic 'the poor man's penicillin', says garlic extract treats *parvovirus*, a disorder that in dogs leads to excessive intestinal bleeding and death.

Top-priced thoroughbreds at the famous Newmarket racing stables in England consume buckets of the stinking rose every day. According to Professor John Heinerman, a world authority on herbs and herbal medicines, breeders found that modern medicines were not always effective against the various diseases that used to cripple the horses. Lord John Fitzgerald was the first of the local trainers to experiment with the bulb. He used it to prevent viruses, eliminate worms and keep the blood thin, which protects the heart.

In Southern Europe, garlic is fed to the horses to increase fertility. It is said "to make the stallions' blood race."

Garlic has had its brush with celebrity pets, as well. When actress June Lockhart started losing the battle with her dog Tony's fleas, she was told to mix garlic extract with his food.

"The flea problem just disappeared," she says. In fact, Lockhart, who became a spokesperson for International Hearing Dog, Inc. after starring in the *Lassie* TV series, was so excited by garlic's powers that she arranged for the extract to be sent out with every newly trained dog.

How to Use Garlic for Your Pet

Although you should try to use fresh, raw garlic whenever possible, granu-

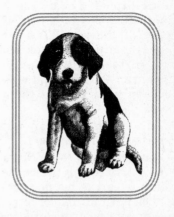

lated or extracts will suffice if you have no choice. Grate a little into your pet's food at every meal – about ½ to 3 cloves – depending on the animal's size.

82

Bland Diets for Mild Stomach Distress

Dogs
4 cups cooked white rice
2 cups low-fat cottage cheese
2 cups boiled or broiled and diced
**   skinless chicken**
¼ clove fresh-pressed garlic

Mix the ingredients well and serve 3-4 times a day. This should provide enough food – more or less – for an average 20-30 pound dog for one day. Once the condition improves, wean the pet back to the regular food over a few days.

Cats
1 cup rice baby cereal
**   (pre-mixed with water)**
1 cup strained turkey,
**   chicken or lamb baby food**
½ cup low-fat cottage cheese
⅛-¼ clove fresh-pressed garlic

Mix ingredients and divide into 3-4 meals.

Dry Skin Supplement for Dogs

1 Tbs corn or safflower oil
1 tsp brewer's yeast
¼ clove fresh-pressed garlic

Mix ingredients and add to food daily.

Vegetarian Diet for Dogs

3 cups boiled white rice
2 Tbs corn or safflower oil
2 large hard-boiled eggs, chopped
¼ tsp calcium carbonate
¼ tsp salt
¼ tsp potassium chloride
½ clove fresh-pressed garlic

Hypoallergenic Diets

Dogs
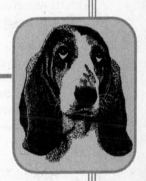
4 oz boiled, diced lamb
2 cups boiled white rice
1 tsp safflower oil
1½ tsp dicalcium phosphate
¼ clove fresh-pressed garlic

Cats
4 oz strained lamb baby food
1 cup rice baby cereal
¾ tsp dicalcium phosphate
¼ clove fresh-pressed garlic

Low-Sodium Diet for Dogs

¼ lb lean ground beef
2 cups boiled white rice without salt
1 Tbs corn or safflower oil
2 tsp dicalcium phosphate
½ clove fresh-pressed garlic

Vets and Vinegar

Veterinarians have found that adding one teaspoon of vinegar to each quart of drinking water helps keep your pet free of fleas and ticks.

And vinegar can be used topically for pets, too. It's a low-cost, highly effective ear rinse for keeping cats', rabbits' and dogs' healthy ears clean, as well as for treating yeast or bacteria-infected ears. Dilute vinegar half and half with water. Either dip a cotton swab into the solution and gently clean the inside of the ear or use a bulb syringe. Warning: Don't pour this into a ruptured eardrum.

If you need a homemade antibacterial cleanser in a hurry, you can dunk the same half-and-half vinegar mixture in a clean cloth to disinfect 'hot spots' and other wounds on cats, dogs or horses.

Vinegar can cool the fires of arthritis and hip dysplasia pain, too. Pour some on a compress and soak your pet's aching joints.

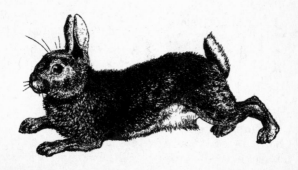

Honey, Kelp & Comfrey

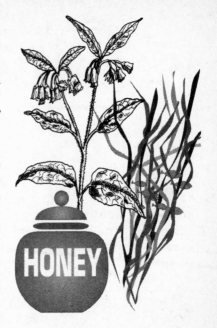

Nature has been good to us, giving us everything we need, if we will only open our eyes and use our heads.

With that in mind, let's look at three natural wonders. They are, in turn, a bee's nectar, a seaweed and an aromatic herb. When you integrate them into a well-balanced diet, they can counteract stress, soothe raw nerves, promote restful sleep, kill bacteria and other germs, stimulate the immune system, increase resistance to cancer and other modern ills, prevent heart disease and disinfect wounds. And that doesn't include their talent for flavoring beverages, desserts, soups, stews and other dishes.

Healthful Honey

Cynics say honey is nothing but a simple sugar, no better than the white powder in your sugar bowl, and only a fool would believe differently.

But what about researchers at the University of Colorado at Boulder, the University of Wisconsin at Madison, Georgetown University Medical Center in Washington, D.C., the Massachusetts Institute of Technology (M.I.T.), Heidelberg University (one of the oldest institutions of higher learning in the Western world) and elsewhere? Scientists at these centers have verified at least one healthful property of honey.

Here are the possible therapeutic benefits of honey:

- **Kills bacteria**
- **Disinfects wounds and sores**
- **Eases the perception of pain**
- **Alleviates asthma**
- **Soothes sore throats**
- **Calms the nerves**
- **Induces sleep**
- **Relieves diarrhea**

Dr. Jarvis says honey is an everyday type of health tonic and recommends it for coughs, sore throats, muscle cramps, burns, stuffy noses, sinusitis, hay fever and other allergies, insomnia and bed-wetting in children.

British researchers have proven that applying honey directly to open wounds keeps them sterile and prevents infections, gangrene and other complications as effectively as any medication known, if not better. In fact, honey can often eliminate the need for conventional (and costly) antibiotics.

Prominent surgeons writing in the prestigious medical journal *The Lancet* say honey-covered wounds heal faster and support less bacterial colonization than wounds treated with ordinary antibiotics. Test-tube experiments showed that honey kills a wide range of infectious microorganisms.

Dr. Jarvis explains why: "It's no mere theory but has been proven that bacteria cannot live in the presence of honey for the reason that honey is an excellent source of potassium."

Subsequent research has suggested that honey may have more going for it than just potassium. Chemical analysis at the University of Wisconsin showed copper, iron and manganese to be present in honey in respectable amounts. Iron, especially, is very important for sustaining the red coloring matter in blood called hemoglobin, which has the task of transporting oxygen to all tissues in the body.

These minerals are present in relatively slight quantities, but experts agree that many minerals are needed by the body in very small amounts to keep the body in balance.

Honey is also rich in vitamin C, riboflavin, nicotinic acid and other B vitamins, which accounts for its widely reported abilities to calm down highly-strung people and to promote a good night's sleep. "A tablespoon of honey at the evening meal makes you look forward to bedtime," writes Jarvis.

Honey is also predigested, reducing the amount of work your stomach has to do before the body can use it. While this is of relatively little importance to healthy individuals, it can mean a great deal to people with impaired digestion.

Here are the advantages of honey:

- **It is non-irritating to the lining of the digestive tract**

- **It is easily and rapidly assimilated**

- **It quickly answers the demand for energy**

- **It helps athletes, laborers and anyone else who expends large amounts of energy to recuperate rapidly from exertion**

- **It places the least strain on the kidneys of all sugars**

- **It has a natural and gentle laxative effect**

- **It has sedative value, quieting the body**

- **It is easily obtainable and widely available**

- **It is inexpensive**

So, doctors might like you to believe honey is no different than white sugar, but don't you believe them.

Honey and Children

"I am saddened when people tell me that they don't eat honey because it costs more than white sugar. I try to make them see that health is not to be had for the asking. Good health is earned. In the long-run, you must pay either the grocer or the druggist.

"When you become sick, you find you must spend the money you saved on food to purchase drugs to bring back your health. By purchasing the right kind of food, such as honey represents, you can constructively cut some corners."

— D.C. Jarvis, MD

Now, how's that for good old-fashioned common sense?

Adding honey to your child's milk will improve its quality.

Jarvis recommends adding one to two teaspoons of honey to eight ounces of milk. "Children fed on honey rarely have colic; the rapid absorption of honey prevents fermentation from taking place," he says.

He believes the potassium it supplies is vital for the rapid growth of a child's body. At the same time, honey is palatable, calming and full of minerals.

Because of the nature of its sugars, honey provides both a quick-energy release and a slow-energy release, which maintains the child's blood glucose level, avoiding the swings and crashes one would see with processed sugar.

Studies at the Universities of Minnesota and Chicago confirmed these observations, and doctors there say honey should be more widely used to maintain your child's health.

CAUTION: The Center for Disease Control says we should not give honey to children under one year of age.
The reason is that botulism bacterial spores stick to honey. In adults, the immune system is mature and strong enough to fight off such attacks. But a child that young is not ready to take on such a powerful foe.

Honey and Bed-Wetting

Bed-wetting is another area in which parents can make good use of honey. While the problem is quite normal in the first three years of life, when it continues well beyond that age, it needs some attention.

And honey, it may surprise you, is an effective, natural, inexpensive and tasty treatment your child will love, Jarvis says.

"At bedtime, give the child a teaspoonful of honey. It will act in two ways. First, it will act as a sedative to the nervous system. Second, it will attract and hold fluid during the hours of sleeping." Try it every night at first until you notice results. Then observe what conditions are likely to produce an episode of bed-wetting. Hold honey in reserve for those occasions, and use it as a preventive treatment.

Try this great honey-based cough remedy: Boil one lemon slowly for 10 minutes. Cut in two and extract the juice with a lemon squeezer (the softened rind and pulp will yield a larger quantity of juice than a lemon straight out of the refrigerator). Pour the juice into a glass or jar and add enough honey so the mixture thickens (if you can obtain glycerin at a pharmacy, add two table-spoons). If you have no lemons, use apple cider vinegar. Take a teaspoon when you wake up, in the middle of the morning, with the midday meal, in the midafternoon, after supper and at bedtime.

Here's another surprising use for honey: At times we're all plagued by an annoying twitching of the eyelids or at the corner of the mouth. To treat it, take two teaspoons of honey at each meal. As a rule, it will disappear within a week's time.

Honey is a remarkable remedy for burns, as well. Apply it directly to steam burns and burns from open flames or hot objects. It relieves the sting-ing and smarting, stops the for-mation of blisters, prevents infection, produces rapid heal-ing and keeps scarring to a minimum.

By the way, honey is a sugar, and if you use too much it can contribute to weight gain. Use it in moderation.

For those of you thinking that honey sounds old-fash-ioned, stop for a minute and think of all the modern reme-dies for burns, blisters, bed-wetting, coughs, cuts, colds,

hayfever and the like. How well do they work? Most doctors will admit not that well. Even when they do work, just read the list of contraindications (risks and hazards) and you'll see that sometimes the treatment may be worse than the cure.

If the fancy explanations don't clear up the mystery of honey, take comfort in the words of Dr. Blodgett, "Who cares why it works? It just does. Honey's got something in it that's clearly very good for you."

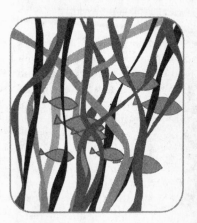

Kelp

Kelp is an old-time word for seaweed. It's powerful stuff.

Modern science confirms that seaweed is an all-around wonder, nutritionally, medical-ly and pharmaceutically.

Here are a few of its astounding health benefits:

- Kills bacteria
- Smothers cancer
- Fortifies the immune system
- Heals ulcers
- Lowers cholesterol levels
- Reduces blood pressure
- Prevents strokes
- Thins the blood

The reason for this expansive talent is simple: Almost every chemical known on earth dissolves in the oceans. This means that plant and animal life growing in the sea are not deficient in any of the elements necessary to support life.

In this day and age, the one drawback to the ocean acting as a depository for all the chemicals on earth is that it collects pollution, toxic wastes and garbage, as well as life-sustaining elements. But most scientists think the benefits of seafood (fish and kelp) outweigh the drawbacks.

Folk medicine users have known for centuries what science is just learning: Kelp is a true health treasure.

An Illustrious History

Throughout history, people have had tremendous luck and great results using kelp to treat constipation, bronchitis, emphysema, asthma, indigestion, ulcers, colitis, gallstones, obesity and disorders of the genitourinary and reproductive systems, both male and female, according to Dr. Varro Tyler, Dean of the School of Pharmacy, Nursing and Health Sciences at Purdue University in Lafayette, IN.

He says that kelp also helps clean out the bloodstream, strengthen disease resistance, quell arthritis and rheumatism discomfort, soothe and calm frayed nerves, counteract stress, and treat many skin diseases, burns and insect bites.

Studies in the past two decades have clearly shown that many of these claims have a firm basis in fact. Kelp contains chemicals that can prevent and treat several types of cancer, curb high cholesterol and high blood pressure (the two prime culprits of heart disease), thin the blood, short-circuit ulcers, kill germs and cure constipation (as a plant is therefore very high in fiber).

Why? No one explains it better than Dr. Jarvis: "When seafood, either plant or animal, is eaten, these minerals are reabsorbed and perform their marvelous chemical functions of regulation and correction. The numerous elements coming from the sea, one of the most important of which is iodine, furnish the final essential link in the balanced diet."

He explains that the most essential mineral elements of body composition, in the order of their apparent importance, are iodine, copper, calcium, phosphorus, manganese, sodium, potassium, magnesium, chlorine and sulfur. All of these except iodine, which is a native of the sea, have their source in the soil. We would naturally suppose that when we eat products of the soil we should secure an ample supply of them. That is, no doubt, what nature intended.

But nature did not foresee that man would remove the trees and other growth, allowing the rains to erode the soil. This leeches out the essential minerals and, by means of our creeks and rivers, carries them down to the sea. The result is mineral-poor soil, which produces mineral-poor food. Stresses Jarvis: "The obvious result is that humans, who depend upon these mineral-starved foods for our supply of minerals, are literally starving in the midst of plenty."

The long and short of this is that when somebody tells you vitamin and mineral supplements are unnecessary – that a 'balanced diet' supplies everything you need – they are wrong. That would be true if the land and soil were still at full strength, but we have weakened it. The soil in turn has yielded flimsy food, which is slowly wilting our vitality.

Kelp and Cancer

The Japanese eat vast quantities of seaweed. Epidemiologists have noted that Japanese women have a mere fraction of the breast cancers American women develop; and Japanese women who do fall prey to breast cancer live longer than American or British women with the disease.

The scientists wondered if there was a connection between high seaweed consumption and breast cancer protection. Dr. Jane Teas of the Harvard School of Public Health checked out this theory. Her animal experiments showed that the brown seaweed *laminaria* conferred protection against known cancer-causing chemicals.

A 1974 Japanese study showed that not only could kelp prevent the development of breast cancer, but that it could also treat existing tumors. Kelp slowed the progression of breast malignancies in 95 percent of test animals. Sixty-six percent of them went into complete remission.

Dr. Teas speculates that the chemical called *fucoidan* in seaweed may play a large role in the anti-cancer capacity of kelp, but she notes that seaweeds also have potent antibiotic properties. That means seaweed may have promise in preventing or treating colon cancer, too.

A study at the University of Hawaii School of Medicine in Honolulu showed that a health food popular in Japan, a dried version of the seaweed, *wakame*, helped cure and prevent lung cancer when injected into laboratory animals.

Researchers there found evidence that active ingredients in the seaweed activate the immune system.

Scientists have isolated blood pressure-lowering (hypotensive) chemicals, including histamine, in kelp. Seaweed appears to act as an antidote to excess sodium consumption and may well help prevent strokes.

Kelp tablets are available in many health food stores, as are packaged seaweeds for cooking purposes. A single kelp tablet per day will give you all the minerals you need.

Comfrey

The herb is so potent that it is best for external applications, although it sometimes figures in recipes for healing teas.

Comfrey is recommended for:

- **Healing wounds**
- **Disinfecting cuts**
- **Reducing bruises**
- **Shrinking phlebitis and venous clots**
- **Smoothing wrinkles**
- **Soothing respiratory ailments**
- **Easing digestive ills**

The name 'comfrey' is derived from the Latin word *confervere*, which means to heal or knit together. It has also been called bruisewort, knitbone and healing herb.

Comfrey belongs to the borage family of plants. It is found in damp environments and is native to Europe, western Siberia and the British Isles. It grows to a height of three to four feet, has long, oval leaves covered with sticky hairs, clusters of bell-shaped flowers and a bulbous root.

Beware: Comfrey can easily be confused with foxglove, a mistake that can be serious, or on occasion, even fatal.

Comfrey is available in seed or live plant form.

Researchers report that comfrey ointments or poultices heal almost any kind of sore, bruise or scrape. It also works wonders on insect bites and burns. To make an ointment, mix the powdered comfrey into any soft-based salve such as petroleum jelly, lanolin, wax, butter or lard.

You can also prepare a poultice, a dampened cloth topped with the herb that is spread over the affected area. Sometimes, as with mustard plasters, you'll want to place the herb between two dampened sheets to prevent any falling onto bare skin, which can cause irritation.

For simple cuts, soak comfrey leaves in hot water and apply directly to the cut. Leave in place for one hour.

Shlomo Noy, MD, of Tel Aviv University in Israel, recommends a strong comfrey ointment for phlebitis, a blood clot lodged in a leg vein.

As a treatment for wrinkles and a brisk facial splash, apply comfrey lotion morning and night.

Note: Medical anthropologist John Heinerman, Ph.D., cautions that when taken internally in large amounts over a long period of time, comfrey may cause liver damage.

Try These Other Natural Wonders

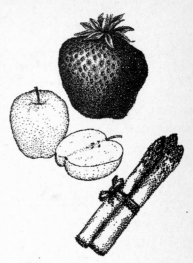

An apple a day won't only keep the doctor away, it can also chase away the blues. A study at Michigan State University revealed that subjects who ate two apples a day had less tension, fewer headaches and less frequent emotional upsets, writes Ben Harris, author of *Home Remedies, Cures and Kitchen Tricks*. And an apple a day will also keep away the dentist. Apples help cleanse teeth of decay-causing carbohydrates, like sugar, and stimulate the gums and saliva flow.

A juice extracted from the roots and lower stems of **asparagus** is said to be an effective kidney remedy. To extract the juice, simply simmer two heaping tablespoons of chopped asparagus roots and lower stems in one quart of hot water for approximately 30 minutes, then strain. Drink a cupful every three to four hours.

Celery is another excellent vegetable for settling nerves, Harris points out. Try the expressed juice of celery leaves and stalks in ½-cup doses, three to four times a day.

The oil from mashed **cloves** can be used for settling nerves of a different sort – in an aching tooth that has lost its filling!

Dates soaked in warm water until cool are said to be a naturally gentle laxative. Chew them well and don't forget to drink the water they were soaking in. A small dose of five or six dates in the morning and at night should be sufficient.

Looking for a first-rate facial? Soak overnight one Tbs of rolled **oats** in two Tbs of buttermilk, then add the beaten white of one egg. Spread over the face and neck and let the mixture settle for 20 to 30 minutes. Remove with a soft washcloth and warm cool water, and repeat twice a day.

Papaya is a wonder fruit. Besides being highly nutritious, it gives immediate relief of indigestion. It also cleans out the intestinal tract and banishes bad breath.

Strawberries are excellent for the teeth. They prevent tartar buildup and dissolve tartar that has already taken hold. Halve the strawberry and rub it over the teeth. Allow the juice to stay on the teeth a minute or two before rinsing.

Here are three herbs you may be less familiar with:

Chamomile
(Anthemis nobilis)

Chamomile flowers, which are so pretty, are also excellent for our health. Chamomile grows wild, especially in meadows, creeping across the surface of the ground, rooting where they want, and dividing into branches and large, close-knit patches.

Chamomile can be purchased in flower, tea bag, tincture, extract or juice form.

It is an absolute wonder herb for digestion. The flowers are prepared in a tea, one or two tablespoons to a cup of boiling water. Drink half a cupful at a time.

Chamomile also helps relieve stomachache in babies and small children. Strain before adding it to a baby bottle, and always use it in a diluted form. It is an ancient remedy for children's diarrhea and a wonderful aid to restful sleep.

It also makes an excellent insect repellent. Splash some chamomile tea on your exposed skin, face, arms and legs, before you go out.

But be warned: Chamomile flowers grow on the ground and are sometimes accidentally picked along with ragweed. If you are allergic to ragweed, be very careful!

Ginger
(Zingiber officinale)

Ginger tea is an excellent aid in preventing colds, says Dr. Buchman. She recommends using a combination of peppermint, a pinch of ginger and a pinch of

clove powder or two bruised cloves. Ginger tea can be used to combat nausea and to stimulate the digestive organs. It grows readily in the garden and is widely available in root form in Oriental groceries and fruit stores.

Grated ginger baths can help ease muscle and joint pain and improves sluggish circulation. Just drop a few granules of grated ginger in the bathtub. Don't use too much. Like cayenne, ginger quickly brings the blood to the surface.

To make ginger tea, use a pinch to a tablespoonful of the powder, or grate or slice the fresh root. Simmer in water until the brew turns yellowish. For pain, soak a cloth or a sponge in ginger tea and apply directly to the area of pain.

Ginseng
(Panax quinquefolia)

Ginseng is an excellent tonic and pick-me-up. Researchers say it sharpens memory, stops coughing, and helps prevent, and fight, colds.

You can buy ginseng as a dried root, a tincture, a powder or an extract.

To restore energy, drop a pinch of ginseng powder in a cup of hot water and drink it. Or you can use a prepared ginseng tea extract, a capsule of powdered root, or chew on a piece of raw root.

Japanese scientists, principally professors S. Shibata and K. Takagi, claim that their experiments on mice proved that ginseng added to the diet increases – and speeds up – the ability to absorb information. And students at Uppsala University in Sweden who added ginseng to their daily diet, studied better, worked faster and scored consistently higher on tests than their peers.

Most of the peoples of the Far East use ginseng to treat a whole range of illnesses – from the common cold to arthritis, respiratory ailments like bronchitis and asthma, and inflammation of all kinds. Enthusiasts chew it as a root, add the powder to their tea, and use the extract in drinks and food.

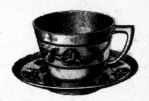